MEDITATE AND BE MADE WHOLE
THROUGH JESUS CHRIST

Printed and bound in Great Britain by
CPI Antony Rowe, Chippenham and Eastbourne

Published by Crossbridge Books
Tree Shadow, Berrow Green
Martley WR6 6PL
Tel: +44 (0)1886 821128   www.crossbridgebooks.com
© Crossbridge Books 2009

First published 2009

ISBN 978-0-9561787-1-8

British Library Cataloguing in Publication Data.
A catalogue record for this book is available from
the British Library.

Also by Trevor Dearing (available from the publisher):

It's True!
The God of Miracles Trevor and Anne Dearing
Total Healing
God and Healing of the Mind
Always Here for You

BIBLICAL QUOTATIONS
unless otherwise shown, are from the Holy Bible, New International Version
used with permission.

MEDITATE AND BE MADE WHOLE THROUGH JESUS CHRIST

REV. TREVOR DEARING M.A. B.D.

A Biblical Manual for Divine Healing

CROSSBRIDGE BOOKS

Preface

I have written eleven books previous to this one. My writing began with the publication of my book "Wesleyan and Tractarian Worship" in 1966, setting forth the common factors in the worship of John Wesley and the Tractarian movement which began the High Church Catholic Movement in the Church of England. There was an interval in my writing until I wrote the book "Exit the Devil" in 1976. This related the story of my own conversion and miraculous healing, followed later by my baptism in the Holy Spirit on May 10th 1969 and the beginning of my ministry at St Paul's Hainault in 1970. The book told of how the Holy Spirit made a wonderful supernatural visitation not only to myself and later to my wife Anne, but also to what had been a small church down Arrowsmith Road on the Hainault housing estate on the outskirts of London.

Eventually at least 600 people gathered at that church every Tuesday evening for our "Power, Praise and Healing Services", wherein the Lord used me and my helpers in bringing about hundreds of conversions and miraculous healings. The church, with myself, became the focus of mass media attention both in England and other parts of the world, for many came from overseas, and indeed many many lives were changed and miraculously transformed by the Holy Spirit during my ministry at St Paul's 1970 -75.

In 1976 I described all these events in "Exit the Devil",

published in England, selling many hundreds of copies and resulting in great interest in what had now become the itinerant ministry of myself and my wife around the UK and the world.

Our ministry came to the attention of Logos International in America, and I conducted four Conventions of the Holy Spirit for them in Jerusalem and later in Switzerland. They asked me to write for their book publishing department, and so in 1977 I wrote "Supernatural Superpowers" which was a Biblical study about the existence of the Devil, his minions and his occult kingdom; the victory of Christ over them and how God had brought into being a Spirit-filled church which could, in His name, overcome the evil force and so further His kingdom here on earth by driving them from human lives and even nations.

This was followed in 1979 by another book, published by Logos called "Supernatural Healing Today", which was a study of the Divine healing ministry based on Biblical principles and depicting how ministers and churches could enter the realm of Divine healing.

In 1981 Anne and I took over the pastorship of St Luke's Episcopal Church in Seattle where we had a wonderful ministry in the Holy Spirit, but I suffered a "burn-out". However, Bridge Publishers, who had bought out Logos, published a book of mine called "God and Healing of the Mind" which set out the principles of the Biblical basis for the healing of the emotions as well as the mind. It was a manual also for counsellors and depicted a way in which believers who were suffering psychiatric and emotional problems could themselves find healing. After I returned to England in 1983, Marshall Pickering published a book of mine entitled "A People of Power" (1985) in which I showed how a Spirit-anointed pastor and Spirit-anointed Christians should minister and work together in harmony and power in a renewed church. In

1996 Mohr Books, publishers who later took over as Crossbridge Books, published my book entitled "It's True!" which set forth the story of my life and ministry until the leaving of America, thus bringing the account of my ministry up to date. They also published "Total Healing", which elucidated and furthered the teaching about Divine healing given in "Supernatural Healing Today" which had gone out of print.

In 2004 Crossbridge Books published "The God of Miracles" which included the testimonies of large numbers of thankful people, giving details of cases of healing brought about by Jesus of an immensely vast range of illnesses (144) through the ministry of Anne and myself. These were medically verified and long lasting and the book has proved an inspiration to many who have wondered about this ministry and whether they themselves could be healed. Crossbridge Books published a new edition of "God and Healing of the Mind" in 2006 and also a book entitled "Always here for you" in 2007, a small pocket-size book where I used the parable of the Good Samaritan to show how from before our birth we could be robbed by the enemy's powers and the enemy's robbeis, stealing our peace. I went on to show how Christians could find healing from the hurts, bruises and storms of life. This present book is a deeper and more enlarged teaching of this latter publication and I hope it will help people who believe on the Lord Jesus Christ and who are suffering, to find healing through meditation on the Word of God.

PSALM 1

Blessed is the man
   who does not walk in the
     counsel of the wicked
       or stand in the way of sinners
   or sit in the seat of mockers,
But his delight is in the Law of the LORD,
   and on his Law he meditates
     day and night.
He is like a tree planted by streams of water
   which yields its fruit in season
   and whose leaf does not wither.
   Whatever he does prospers.

Not so the wicked!
   They are like chaff
     that the wind blows away.
   Therefore the wicked will not stand
     in the judgment,
     nor sinners in the assembly
       of the righteous.

For the LORD watches over the way
   of the righteous,
but the way of the wicked will perish.

Acknowledgements

I would like to acknowledge the tremendous help of my wife of 51 years, Anne, who has been more than a helpmeet to me but also a partner in spiritual growth and powerful ministry. She has always been an encourager and an inspiration even at times when I myself may have been a bit down. I could not have ever envisaged life without her and in particular my supernaturally anointed ministry, without her being by my side.

I would like to thank Keith Barwell of St George's Church, Stamford, for the equipment on which to record this book and special thanks to May Lloyd, Pastor at Stamford Free Church (Baptist) who has taken the trouble to type this book ready for the publisher.

I would not like to close these acknowledgements without thanking my loyal and faithful publisher Eileen Mohr, who has encouraged me to write books, and has published them. She is not only a publisher, but has been a follower and encourager of my ministry since St Paul's Hainault 1971-75. She wrote at the end of "The God of Miracles" the following testimony: "We owned a 12 seater Land-Rover at the time of hearing what was happening at St Paul's Hainault every Tuesday evening, so I found myself frequently transporting people from Harlow to Hainault who were seeking healing. By the time Trevor's ministry there came to an end I counted up how many people I had taken there. I remembered 31. Of that number, with the exception of one lady whom I did not know well and with whom I did not keep in contact, each had been healed." So my publisher is not publishing these books of mine and my wife Anne out of a sort of blindness of hope that they convey the truth. She herself, as a devoted Christian, has an intense interest in the Divine healing ministry, has been used in it, has witnessed many of the events described, and has proved many of the teachings which I have put in my books to be trustworthy and to actually work in the lives of those whom she has known. Our ministry of healing has proved that miracles of healing can be experienced by anyone, even if they are a bit sceptical. I hope that as you read this book you will find the wholeness which is God's perfect will for all His people.

Contents

Introduction

My wife has a short poem which she often recites to me. One of the verses goes like this:

"We live in an age of getting, of always demanding more
And then when we get it, we're still not contented,
Of this I am certain and sure."

That, in my experience, has certainly been true of the age in which we live. Another sign of the age we live in is the way in which the pace of life in our society has phenomenally increased. This is in spite of the fact that there are more labour-saving devices, scientific and technological innovations together with fewer working hours and longer holidays. Still people in our modern culture want everything to come to them very rapidly. Patience is in very short supply today, as we find often when we are driving and hesitate for a little while to find our way, only to be greeted with blasts of the horn behind us. People want everything at the press of a button; instantaneously. This is also true, in our experience, of the ministry of Divine healing.

Our book, The God of Miracles, covers a hundred and forty-four different illnesses and medical conditions which have been healed in the Name of Jesus through the ministry of Anne and myself down the years. Many of these miracles involve several different people and very rarely is it just one person who has been healed of a particular complaint. Healing, as I indicate in the book, has come through various Biblical ways of healing in the

Name of Jesus. These have been healings through the laying on of hands; the use of the voice in spoken words into people's lives and situations and illnesses, or the word of knowledge, whereby the healing minister knows by Divine revelation what is exactly the problem of health in a person in his congregations and can assure that he or she will be healed, without having to be told by that person initially what their condition actually is. We have also used the spoken word in an authoritative manner as did Jesus and the Apostles, always in the name and under the authority of our Lord and for His glory.

People have also been "born again" or healed through the preaching of God's word. Our ministry of petition and intercession in prayer has perhaps taken some time of faithful prayer before the person has been healed. However, as the book The God of Miracles shows, people have personally testified on many occasions to instantaneous healing; although a lot of cases have been where the healing has begun dramatically at the time of the ministry but taken probably a few days to come to fruition. There is only one case in the Bible which I see as not absolutely instantaneous and where Jesus himself had to minister to a person twice. This is in the healing of the blind man as recorded in Mark chapter 8 verses 22-26 where the blind man was partially healed at the first ministry and fully healed at the second.

So when we minister to the sick we are believing for instantaneous healing. However, we have to concede that, if Jesus had to minister on two occasions, so might we, fallible and imperfect human channels, have to minister to a person on more than one occasion. Also, in our experience whereas the healing has begun at the time of ministry, it has indeed often taken time and patience on the part of the receiver to fully enter into the prayer which we uttered and the ministry which we gave him or her at a particular time.

I am sure, from considerable experience, that many people come to our healing services quite unprepared spiritually to receive the healing from the Lord Jesus at our hands. They also want instantaneous healing at that very moment of ministry and if it is not forthcoming they often go away feeling disillusioned or that "it didn't work for me", or "God doesn't really want to heal me", or simply "it just doesn't work". I feel very sad that this is very often the attitude of people. For I am sure that if they kept faith, they would receive healing after a short time. We have even known of cases where people have felt worse for a few days after the ministry, before waking up one morning and finding that they have in fact been healed.

The way I am going to show how to receive God's healing through Jesus Christ in this book is not in any way to be looked upon as an instantaneous miracle, although in fact, such may rarely occur. I am asking you through the teaching of this book to have patience. I am asking you to give God time and space in your life to quite a sacrificial extent, but I am sure you can find this time and space if you are eagerly and expectantly wishing to receive healing and, for instance, if you are in considerable pain.

This teaching I am about to set forth in the following pages is how to obtain God's healing through meditation. I want to say right at the outset that this is not "transcendental meditation" which is practised in some Eastern religions or even by mystical Christians in Christianity. In such meditation the person at prayer seeks to empty their mind of absolutely every thought and concept and fasten their spirit and soul onto the transcendental Being who is thought of as without attributes or desires but is simply an empty but nevertheless a meaningful void in the mind which the soul fastens onto. I am not going to teach you about meditating the way that is practised in Buddhism, Hinduism or any other religion including Islam. This is going to be exclusively CHRISTIAN MEDITATION which is meditation not in any void, but specifically on the word of God, the Bible. It is this Word which will bring us healing, for it is God's Word, not only to the human race but to every individual living and especially to His believing children who are part of His family, part of His Kingdom, and I believe, He wishes to heal.

So, have patience, *do* what I suggest to you in this book, especially in the meditational exercises. Give it your all: body, mind and spirit, and I believe that as you wait upon the Lord, as Isaiah says, you *"will renew your strength"* and not only that, you will receive what St Paul describes as *"the peace that transcends all understanding"*, and as you receive the word of God into your very being with expectancy and longing you will also receive healing of your body.

Chapter One

The Heart of Meditation

Since my conversion, at the age of nineteen, I have had very wide Christian experience and exposure to every kind of Christian expression in every kind of church except the Brethren. From the age of 19 I was a Methodist and I learned the riches of Methodist theology and Methodist devotion. My experience at the Methodist Bible college. Cliff College, Derbyshire, brought me to an intense realisation of the importance and truth of the Bible in Christian life, worship, and devotion. I especially appreciated the sung theology of Charles Wesley's hymns and, eventually, at Wesley College, Headingley , Leeds, I had a very rich, deep, and wide theological education, culminating in my obtaining a Bachelor of Divinity degree. I then went out into Methodist circuit ministry and appreciated the deep fellowship which is one of the riches of the Methodist Church. However, as my own spiritual life developed from what had been nothing, I became far more sacramental in my theology and wanted the sacrament of Holy

Communion to be at the heart of my Christian worship and devotion, with that of my wife Anne. I therefore went into the Church of England ministry and had a year at Queens College, Birmingham where I continued to study, especially Christian worship, and wrote my thesis, 'Wesleyan and Tractaiian worship'. However, the emphasis on personal devotion was much richer and deeper than it had been at Wesley College Headingley. I was taught to appreciate not only the value of liturgical worship, but also great emphasis was put on the life of personal devotion. Here I learned the value of SILENCE and I was taught how to meditate by Canon Arthur Gribble, the principal, and also the value of auricular confession and how to make a good confession. Eventually, as an Anglican vicar, I found this emphasis in my personal devotional life to be very rich. So when we became itinerant ministers in 1975 I was invited to preach not only in Anglican churches, but also in Roman Catholic seminars and prayer meetings, Pentecostal, Baptist, Methodist and Independent churches, and in fact every Christian denomination.

So my Christian experience and fellowship became very wide and I learned to appreciate all the different emphases of these different expressions of Christian worship and devotion. My baptism in the Holy Spirit on May 10th 1969 came about through my sharing the riches of the Pentecostal Church's emphasis on the Holy Spirit, and eventually this led my wife and myself into our ministry of Divine Healing and teaching worldwide. What I learned at Queens College about the devotional life has continued to be an essential part of my Christian pilgrimage. So prayer has been at the heart of my spiritual devotions and especially the use of silence and exercising the Biblical emphasis on meditation.

This brings me to the very important matter as to whether or not meditation is really a Christian expression of devotion, since it has been widely used by other religions than the Christian. For this reason some Christians are suspicious about it. However, it has to be said that other religions also have prayer at the heart of their faith and Christians do not stop praying because other religions use the avenue of prayer to reach their god or gods. So too, with meditation. Because other religions use the practice of meditation in various ways it does not mean to say that this spiritual discipline is not an essential part of a Christian's spiritual life. Indeed, for me it has been the heart of my Christian devotion. It is not a matter as to whether one prays or not or meditates or not. It is to whom one prays that is of fundamental importance and indeed, as we shall see, it is upon what one meditates that is of vital importance for specifically Christian meditation.

Christian meditation has its roots deeply in the Word of God. It is mentioned quite a lot in the Bible; for instance, Joshua in chapter 1 v 8 commanded his people that they should meditate on the Law of God day and night. Before this, the Bible records in Genesis chapter 24 verse 63 that Isaac went out to meditate in the fields. However for me, the Psalter portrays the heart of Hebrew and therefore also Christian devotions. There in that book of psalms are recorded the prayers and hymns of the Old Testament people which were inherited by the Christians and became part of Christian devotion, as they still are to this day. The psalmist in Psalm 1 v 2 says, *"on His law he* [the good man] *meditates day and night".* In Psalm 63 v 6 the psalmist says, *"I will meditate on Thee in the night watches".* In Psalm 77 v 12 the psalmist says, *"I will meditate also on all thy works"* and in Psalm 143 v 5 this is repeated when the psalmist says, *"I meditate on all thy works".* The word 'meditate' in Hebrew *haggah* is not always translated 'meditate' in new translations of the Bible, but this is what it really means. Psalm 119 is full of the devotees to Yahweh talking about

3

the fact that they will meditate (see Psalm 119 v 15, 119 v 23, 119 v 48, 119 v 78, 119 v 148). Paul urges Timothy to meditate upon the things of God as recorded in 1 Tim 4 v 15 (KJV). The riches of the spiritual life being deepened through meditation are again recorded in the Psalms, in Psalm 49 v 3 and in Psalm 5 v 1. In Psalm 19 v 14 the psalmist says: *"May the ... meditation of my heart be pleasing in Your sight"* and in Psalm 104 v 34 the psalmist says, *"May my meditation be pleasing to Him"*. Meditation as recorded by the psalmist is not just a short exercise in devotion which is a minor part in spiritual life for the Hebrews, because in Ps 119 v 97 the psalmist cries out: *"Oh, how I love Your law! I meditate on it all day long"*. In Psalm 119 v 99 the psalmist says: *"for I meditate on Your statutes"*.

Thus we see that the practice of meditation is essentially Biblical, part of Hebrew devotion in its essence, and this practice was also inherited by the Christians, who were in the beginning all Jews. They worshipped at the Temple where the book of Psalms was the hymn book of the temple, as it was also recited in the synagogues. So we can take it for granted that the early Christians took meditation seriously and practised it. And ever since the early Church, right though 2000 years it has been the core of Christian devotion.

What then is meditation? It is more than reading the Bible even in a disciplined way. It almost goes without saying that every Christian should read their Bible regularly and get to know its contents intimately. It is best to follow a definite scheme of Bible reading. I, for instance, follow the Church of England lectionary as it is written in the Book of Common Prayer, especially the new versions of the book. This course of Bible reading takes one through the Old Testament, the Gospels, Acts, the Letters and the Book of Revelation in a disciplined manner of reading throughout the whole year. It is important before we begin to meditate that we know our Bibles well. Meditation is also more than Bible study, when we read the Bible either in groups, or led by a Bible teacher, or as individuals, to really understand a particular passage or even chapter of the Bible, comparing scripture with scripture and in going into the depths of this meaning. This should be, again, a part of every Christian's life and indeed church life also. Meditation is really a DEEP PRAYERFUL REFLECTION ON ANYTHING WHICH SPEAKS TO A PERSON ABOUT GOD.

. This deep reflection, done very quietly and in a relaxed manner, brings us closer to God as we enter into deep communion with Him and in fact hear Him speaking to us through the particular meditation which we are undertaking. It is a rich source of spiritual growth in every conceivable way.

In general, this prayerful reflection can be, for instance, on the world of nature and on creation itself. Thus we read about Isaac that he was out in the fields in the evening engaging in meditation when he saw the camels coming carrying his future wife. We can indeed go for walks in the countryside, sit down on a grassy hill, for instance, and view from a height a scene which is before us consisting perhaps of trees, hills, mountains, flowers and so on. I believe that the hymn translated by Stuart K Hine (author unknown) is obviously the result of a deep meditation on the world of nature. He writes

> O Lord my God, when I in awesome wonder
> Consider all the works Thy hand hath made;
> I see the stars, I hear the mighty thunder,
> Thy power throughout the Universe displayed;
> Then sings my soul, my Saviour God, to Thee,

How great Thou art! How great Thou art!
Then sings my soul, my Saviour God, to Thee,
How great Thou art! How great Thou art!
When through the woods and forest glades I wander
And hear the birds sing sweetly in the trees;
When I look down from lofty mountain grandeur,
And hear the brook and feel the gentle breeze
Then sings my soul, my Saviour God, to Thee,
How great Thou art! How great Thou art!

I am sure that Psalm 23, "The Lord is my Shepherd, I shall not want" comes from David's deep reflection on the relationship between himself as a shepherd and the sheep for which he was responsible and for which he was caring. It has of course been a rich source of blessing and consolation for Christians throughout the generations.

So we can go out into God's creation and marvel at it and spend time deeply reflecting upon all its beauty leading us to the Creator Himself. And this can be a rich source of devotional enrichment which can lead us to the heart of God. We can also meditate on hymns, like the one I have quoted above. In Holy Week I spend the whole week meditating on the hymn

"When I survey the wondrous cross
On which the Prince of Glory died"

I take the whole hymn verse by verse and once again I would point out that this hymn, by Isaac Watts, is the result of deep meditation on the cross. This is especially portrayed in the words "when I *survey*". In other words he was in his heart and in his imagination at the hill of Golgotha or Calvary and literally seeing Jesus hanging there upon the cross as he says:

> See from his head, his hands, his feet
> Sorrow and love flow mingled down
> Did e'er such love and sorrow meet
> Or thorns compose so rich a crown?

This hymn, again, has obviously been a rich treasure of devotion for Christians down many years, especially at Passiontide.

Meditation like this involves the whole person: body, mind and spirit. We cannot meditate when we are physically tense because this hinders the whole condition of our being when we are seeking to focus our minds. To meditate we must be physically relaxed. Obviously, like Isaac, we can be very relaxed in mind and soul when we are taking a leisurely walk through the world of nature at any time. However, it is usual to set aside about 20 minutes a day for meditation.

We need a quiet room where we will not in any way be interrupted. We need to sit on a comfortable chair and relax our whole body. A helpful way of doing this which is medically proven, as well as spiritually beneficial, is to take say 20 deep breaths. We breathe in through the nose very deeply, feel our abdomen swell as we put our hand on it and then we exhale through the mouth starting at 20 and counting down to zero. Perhaps our hands are placed on our knees or thighs or we simply lie back in an easy chair which is comfortable and relax our bodies. Then our eyes are very important as we meditate on a hymn or on a passage of scripture (which we shall look at later) and digest it through the eyes. Focusing through the eyes is for most people actually more vivid in its impression on the mind than hearing through the ears. So we see that if we are in a room wanting to concentrate, a television is more of a distraction than a radio. So we **look**. Then we use the faculties of our mind to ingest mentally the subject on which we are meditating. However, the use of sanctified imagination is also very important, as indeed we see in the hymn "When I survey the wondrous cross", for no doubt Isaac Watts was imagining himself there looking at Jesus suffering there in agony for us. We let our minds go free and our imagination also. And rove around whatever it will as long as it is related to the subject on which we are meditating. We must bring all wandering thoughts into captivity very gently to refocus ourselves on the subject of our meditation. This, as I have said, needs to go on for at least 20 minutes, and we shall certainly need to return to the same subject of our meditation over and over again for a week or sometimes even a month until we feel it has become 'stale' to our reflection and penetration and has served its purpose for us.

A former international cricketer, who has now gone to Glory, taught me a practice of what he called 'RELAXED CONCENTRATION'. He said that when he went out to bat for his country, if he was too tense then the delicate strokes or even formidable ones which he needed to play to score runs would not come because he was too tense; his arms and wrists were not flexible enough. On the other hand, if he was too relaxed he would very soon be 'out' as a batsman and back in the pavilion, finished through carelessness. What he had to learn was how to be relaxed and deeply concentrated both at the same time. This took practice.

If a reader is not familiar with this, my favourite sport, then we can see the same necessity for relaxed concentration in that of a concert pianist. If the pianist is too tense then his or her fingers will not move lightly and properly over the keys of the piano, he will make mistakes and the music will not flow. If, again, he is too relaxed he will hit false notes and the whole thing become a mess. Like a cricketer, the pianist has to learn the art of relaxed concentration. This is a necessity in a fruitful meditation. This relaxed concentration is vital, because if we are too tense our imagination and mind will not flow over the subject of our meditation but will wander all over the place. The same would happen if we were too careless and relaxed. We need to be relaxed and concentrated both at the same time. In fact I have found this attitude or condition of relaxed concentration not only to be important in meditation but also for my whole walk with the Lord every minute of the day in my Christian life.

In his book on prayer which has a subtitle of "Finding the heart's true home", Richard Foster tells the story of Jim Smith, a former student of his, who decided to go to a retreat house for a time of silence and to renew his spiritual life.

The author tells of how Jim met a brother who gave him only one assignment: to meditate on the story of the Annunciation in the first chapter of Luke's gospel. Richard Foster then graphically describes the struggle Jim had to come to grips for a whole week with this one scriptural assignment and how to meditate on this passage. It took him some time to find out what the brother was really seeking for him and how to meditate not simply by reading and re-reading the passage, or deeply studying it, but reading it with his *heart*. Richard Foster's whole book, published by Hodder and Stoughton, together with his book, Celebration of Discipline, is really a must for those who wish to study the subject of meditation more widely than I am describing here. However, I feel I have revealed the very heart of meditation in the above description and given anyone enough material and insight in order to start or deepen their meditative life.

The above is a description of meditation in general, but the particular object in writing the present book for the reader is my desire to lead him or her into the practice of meditating on Holy Scripture. This I believe will bring as its uttermost goal a deeper communion with God and thereby a deeper peace, but will also bring wholeness not only to the spirit but also to the mind and body. In fact we shall meditate and find that we are healed. To this specific subject of meditating on the word of God we must now turn by studying how the word of God, the Bible, has within itself the ability, through the action of the Holy Spirit, to bring us wholeness.

Chapter Two

The All-powerful Word

The God in whom Christians believe does not exist in a sort of solitary bliss containing Himself within Himself and having no interest in the human race or individuals in particular. The God in whom Christians believe actually expresses Himself – reveals Himself – He *speaks*. This speech of God is called His LOGOS – His WORD. Ultimately this expression of God, this revelation of Himself, this Word is the most powerful force that exists in all Creation. So the Bible itself speaks about the power of God's word. It teaches that He actually spoke this Universe into existence and it was a word from Him that set the sun ablaze. So the first chapter of the book Genesis, which describes Creation, continually says "God said ..." (for instance, 'Let there be light, and there was light' Genesis chapter 1 verse 2). Peter also says, *"by God's word the Heavens existed and the earth was formed"* (2 Peter chapter 3 verse 5) and the writer of the Letter to the Hebrews says that Jesus sustains *"all things by His powerful word'"* (Hebrews chapter 1 verse 3). In other words, if God stopped speaking, everything would fall into chaos and even cease to exist. So we can set no limits whatsoever on the power of God's word to achieve what He desires.

The Bible teaches that God has revealed His very NAME to the human race. This He did to Moses, as is written in Exodus chapter 3 that Moses actually asked God His name and God said to Moses: "I AM WHO I AM. This is what you are to say to the Israelites: 'I AM has sent me to you'." This is the meaning of the name transliterated 'YAHWEH' or 'JEHOVAH'. Also the name of God in Genesis chapter 2 is given as 'ELOHIM'. So God revealed HIS name firstly to Moses, then to the people of the Hebrews, then to the human race as a whole.

God's word, His revelation, His expression of himself, was actually given to individuals in the Old Testament. So Jeremiah chapter 37 v 6 says: *"Then the word of the LORD came to Jeremiah the prophet"*. This means that the utterance Jeremiah was to make came not from within his own thoughts or consciousness but from outside himself.

In the New Testament the word of the Lord is identified with the person of Jesus. This is especially taught in John's gospel chapter 1. We read: *"In the beginning was the Word, and the Word was with God, and the Word was God. He was with God in the beginning. Through Him all things were made: without Him nothing was made that has been made. In Him was life, and that life was the light of men. The light shines in the darkness, but the darkness has not understood it."* (John chapter 1 verses 1-5) Then comes the startling announcement in John's gospel, chapter 1 verse 14: *"The Word became flesh and made his dwelling among us. We have seen His glory, the glory of the One and Only, who came from the Father, full of grace and truth."*

Later John the Baptist testifies concerning Jesus. He cries out, saying: *"This was He of whom I said, 'He who comes after me has surpassed me because He was before me'."* (See verse 30.) *"From the fulness of his grace we have all received one blessing after another. For the law was given through Moses; grace and truth came through Jesus Christ."* (John chapter 1 v 14 –17)

This teaching is reiterated in the Letter to the Hebrews. Chapter 1 reads: *"In the past God spoke to our forefathers through the prophets at many times and in various ways, but in these last days He has spoken to us by His Son, whom He appointed heir of all things, and through whom He made the Universe. The Son is the radiance of God's glory and the exact representation of His being, sustaining all things by his powerful word."* (Hebrews chapter 1 verses 1-3a.)

So every word and action of Jesus and His person in Himself is, as we read in the Gospels, all that God has spoken – fulfilled and enshrined in Jesus. This revelation of the Word is enshrined in Scripture, which Christians rightly call 'THE WORD OF GOD'.

The Bible, the Scriptures, are regarded by Christians as the CANON OF 'TRUTH; this means they are the rule by which Christians can believe and should act. The Scriptures, as we have them, were inspired by God. This is stated quite unequivocally in Paul's Second Letter to Timothy chapter 3 verses 14-17:

"But as for you, continue in what you have learned and have become convinced of, because you know those from whom you learned it and how from infancy you have known the Holy Scriptures, which are able to make you wise for salvation through faith in Christ Jesus. All Scripture is God-

breathed [inspired] and is useful for teaching, rebuking, correcting and training in righteousness, so that the man of God may be thoroughly equipped for every good work." So we Christians believe that God has spoken in the Old Testament and that this is inspired by Him in every word as originally given. We also extend this to the New Testament which in Jesus and all the rest of the New Testament goes on to speak of God's action, interpreting Christ's life, death and resurrection as inspired. Jesus himself quoted the Old Testament in, for example, the Sermon on the Mount in Matthew chapter 5 where he says, "It has been written" and also in such quotations that we have when Jesus says, as recorded in Matthew 12 v 40, *"For as Jonah was three days and three nights in the belly of a huge fish, so the Son of Man will be three days and three nights in the heart of the earth."*

This canon was formulated, including the New Testament, over a period of many years. Eventually it was accepted by the Church as inspired and the Church believed that through Scripture God speaks today. So every utterance, saying or prophecy (See I Corinthians chapter 12) or revelation or speech made by man in such things as sermons has to be tested by the Bible. God has spoken and still speaks in different ways, but in the end it is the Bible which is now for us the Word of God to our hearts.

Further to the Bible's teaching about the POWER of God's words we also see how the Scriptures teach us about the PERMANENCE OF HIS UTTERANCE. It endures for all ages. Isaiah expresses this truth when he says:

'   *"The grass withers and the flowers fall,*
    But the word of our God stands forever."

(Isaiah chapter 40 verse 8)

and:

14

"so is my word that goes out from my mouth:
it will not return to me empty,
but will accomplish what I desire
and achieve the purpose for which I sent it."

(Isaiah 55 verse 11)

Jesus himself said, *"Heaven and earth will pass away, but my words will never pass away."* (Matthew chapter 24 verse 35)

So we have seen the **power** of God's word, the **permanence** of God's word and also the **purpose** of God's word, which is to accomplish that which God desires.

However, for our study, it is very important to understand, grasp hold of, and never forget the PENETRATION of God's word. So the writer to the Hebrews states:

"The word of God is living and active. Sharper than any double-edged sword, it penetrates even to the dividing of soul and spirit, joints and marrow".

(Hebrews chapter 4 verse 12)

This promises that once the word of God has, as it is able to do, reached the very depths of our being, then it is alive and active within us, doing God's work in our spirits, souls and bodies. So, for instance, if we swallow a medication prescribed by our doctor, it usually contains a chemical substance which becomes active within our body and can affect our minds and emotions. How much more powerful then is the living and active word of God when it is at work within us!

Also we must understand that the Word of God can actually heal us: *"He sent forth his word and healed them"*, Psalm 107 verse 20. However, it is especially on the lips of Jesus that we see the **power**, **permanence**, **penetration** and **purpose** of God's word. For example:

"HE SPOKE" to a storm and there was a great calm.

(Mark chapter 4 verse 39)

"HE SPOKE" and Lazarus came back to life.

(John chapter 11 v 43)

Chapter Three

Meditate and Be Healed

As I stated in the introduction all religions practise meditation in one form or another. This is certainly true of Christian denominations, from the Eastern Orthodox Church to Protestant Churches and through to the Roman Catholic Church. In the practice of meditation it has been found useful to use what is called a 'mantra'. This is a repetitive prayer which is constantly said while the suppliant is meditating. In the Eastern Orthodox Church there is used what is called "the Jesus Prayer". This prayer is "O Jesus Christ, Son of the Living God, have mercy on me, a sinner." The person praying is advised to use this prayer constantly, even as often as he or she breathes, to assist their meditation. The Roman Catholics use the rosary as a form of meditation. There are what are called five joyful mysteries, five sorrowful mysteries and there are 'luminous mysteries'.

The actual mysteries used are: the Annunciation (Luke chapter 1 verses 26-38); the visitation of the Virgin Mary to Elizabeth (Luke chapter 1 vv 39-56); the Nativity itself (Luke chapter 2 verses 1-20); the presentation of Christ in the Temple (Luke chapter 2 verses 21-39); and the finding of the Child Jesus in the Temple (Luke chapter 2 verses 41-52). Those are the joyful mysteries.

The sorrowful mysteries are: Jesus' agony in the Garden of Gethsemane (Luke chapter 22 verses 39-46); the scourging of Jesus (Matthew chapter 27 verse 26); the crowning of Jesus with thorns (Matthew 27 verses 27-31); the carrying of the Cross (John 19 v 17 –18) and the Crucifixion itself (Luke 23 verses 33- 43).

The last Pope added the mysteries of the baptism of Jesus in the Jordan (Luke chapter 3 verses 1-22); the wedding at Cana in Galilee (John chapter 2 verses 1-11); the proclamation of the Kingdom in the Sermon on the Mount (Matthew chapters 5-7); the transfiguration (Mark 9 verses 2 -12) and finally the Last Supper (Matthew chapter 26 verses 17-30).

These meditations and others are practised for their own sake, to bring a person closer to God, for spiritual enrichment and spiritual growth. Our study in this book embraces all this in the word 'wholeness' but we are seeking as a major by-product of meditation to focus our attention on scripture passages, or texts, which speak of wholeness. This means the healing of the spirit, the mind (or soul) and even the body, as with our spirit and our meditation through imagination, the use of the mind and the emotions, we absorb the word of God into our innermost being and are drawn into the very heart of God.

There is a rationale behind all this and not simply sheer guesswork. The fact is that a human being is a 'spiritual, psychosomatic organism'. This means that there is an interaction between spirit, soul and body. Each one affects the other in a very dramatic way. An illustration would be that if we were standing on a road and we suddenly saw a lorry with failed brakes hurtling towards us, we would see the lorry with our eyes (the body). The signal would be flashed to our mind, especially the emotions (the soul), again it would be our mind that would order our body to run for our lives out of the way, and probably we would shoot up an arrow prayer with our spirit that we (and others) might be delivered from this danger. Similarly, if we are physically ill it can affect our emotions and bring about depression, about which again we might pray in our spirit, although even our spiritual relationship with God can be affected by depression. If we are mentally unwell, it can also affect our bodies because something like stress can produce physical effects even in the stomach. So what I am proposing in this book is that if we absorb something through our eyes, i.e. 'the words of Scripture' and meditate upon them with the whole of our soul (our mind, imagination and emotions) and also use our will to keep our minds focused; then there can be effects on the whole of our being. Thus meditation on healing can bring about the healing of our minds and even our bodies. See Figure A, page 22.

For such wholeness to take place and, what we are aiming for also through this meditation, the HEALING OF OUR BODIES, certain fundamental factors have to be part of our approach to such meditation. So, we must without doubt believe that the Bible, on whose words we are meditating, is the inspired word of God. We must believe that the Holy Spirit caused these words to be written; as we have said earlier they are GOD BREATHED. So the Holy Spirit not only inspired the words of the Bible, on which we shall be meditating, but actually uses these words, impregnates these words with His presence. So as we absorb these words into our innermost being and are lifted up in the spirit through meditation, the Holy Spirit will be at work within us, bringing about what the words suggest and in fact promise. So our approach to meditation in order to receive wholeness must be with absolute faith in the Bible as God's word and we must absorb it into our being, "living and active and sharper than any double-edged sword", able to divide between soul and spirit; the very depths of our being. From these depths of our being the healing promised in the meditation will flow out through our spirit into our mind, bringing wholeness there and further into our body, bringing the healing which we so much need.

A mantra is not necessary for Christian meditation, as we shall see in the guided meditations which follow. However the presence and power of the Holy Spirit is essential in our meditation. I find it imperative to ask the Holy Spirit to be present in my meditation and I usually begin with a prayer:

' "For as much as without Thee we are not able to please Thee, ,mercifully grant, O God, that Thy Holy Spirit may in this act of meditation direct and rule my heart through Jesus Christ our Lord."

If I need a mantra at all that is:-"Holy Spirit direct and rule my heart". This indeed helps us to remember the presence and power of God in our meditation and to focus our minds on what we are in fact doing.

I have mentioned above that depression can spoil our communion with God but on the other hand, our meditation itself can bring an end to depression. However there are other impediments to our communion with God in meditation. One of these is pretence (see Luke 18, the parable of the Pharisee and the tax collector). The Pharisee came to God with all the right words but it was actually the tax collector who was real with God and cried out, "Lord have mercy on me, a sinner". Another impediment to our communion with God is unconfessed sin and guilt, and we must make sure we have confessed all our sins to God and as it were, put them under the blood of Christ; in other words, see that Jesus has taken all our sins away by his perfect sacrifice on the Cross. Bitterness and unforgiveness in our hearts can also prevent a real communion with God and we must examine our lives to see that we are not bitter to anyone who has hurt us. Or any circumstances of life which we have found to be distressing and that we do not hold unforgiveness towards anyone who has in fact sinned against us in our lives.

Further impediments are anxiety and fear, legalism in our religion so that we have many lists of prohibitions in our minds when in fact Paul said, "We are not under law but under grace." A sense of inferiority and a complete lack of self-love, negating Jesus' words that we should love our neighbour as ourselves can also be a stumbling block, as can oversensitivity: thinking that people are always criticising us or talking about us or being very sensitive to things which seemingly are said or done against us when they are not. Self pity also has to be avoided and we must make sure we are living a life in obedience to God and not in disobedience in any factor or any way in our daily living. Again there is a prayer in the prayer book which I like to pray and can find no better words myself to help a meditation:

"Almighty God, unto whom all hearts are open, all desires known and from whom no secrets are hid: Cleanse the thoughts of our hearts by the inspiration of Thy Holy Spirit, that we may perfectly love Thee, and worthily magnify Thy Holy Name; through Jesus Christ our Lord. Amen."

So, armed with these prayers, we can begin to meditate upon the word of God and believe for our wholeness as our lives are in a right relationship with God and remember that He has said, *"Come near to .God and He will come near to you"* (James 4 v 8).

So to these meditations upon the word of God we will now turn.

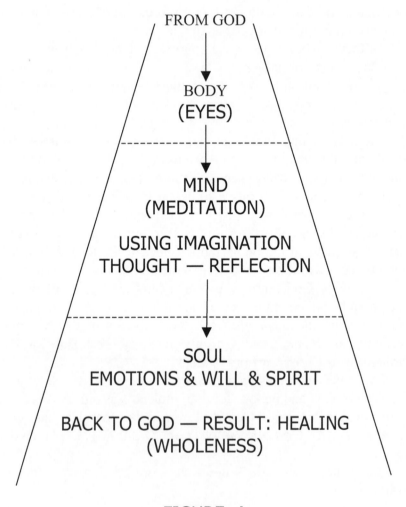

WORD OF GOD
IMPREGNATED BY POWER OF HOLY SPIRIT

FROM GOD

BODY
(EYES)

MIND
(MEDITATION)

USING IMAGINATION
THOUGHT — REFLECTION

SOUL
EMOTIONS & WILL & SPIRIT

BACK TO GOD — RESULT: HEALING
(WHOLENESS)

FIGURE A

Suggested method of how to use
the following verses and passages of Scripture

• I Read this whole book, including the Biblical verses but leaving the meditations until you later select the topics that speak to you, slowly several times. You will find it a manual of Biblical teaching concerning Divine healing, covering a very large range of areas included in this very important subject.

• 2 Note any topic that speaks to you in a special way and use that one to start your discipline of meditation.

• 3 Then re-read the variety of topics and take a second one, then a third, and so on until you have covered them all.

• 4 Before you start each meditation begin with the suggested prayer on page 21, repeating it slowly and making it your own prayer for the guidance of the Holy Spirit during your meditation.

• 5 Memorise each text or passage of Scripture before you actually engage upon it.

• 6 Read my notes, then begin your own meditation until it all comes together as a harmonious whole; the fruit on your own meditation, which may vary from mine.

• 7 Make your own notes in the section provided about what you have heard God say to you and what you have learnt. The whole book will then become your own treasury of devotion.

• 8 You can keep coming back to a particular topic repeatedly as need arises.

• 9 End each meditation by praying the Lord's Prayer.

Meditations arranged according to the order in which they occur in the Bible

A MEDITATION FOR THOSE WHO ARE IN A STATE OF PANIC

Exodus 14 verses 10-13, 21, 22, 25

10*As Pharaoh approached, the Israelites looked up, and there were the Egyptians, marching after them. They were terrified and cried out to the LORD.* 11*They said to Moses, "Was it because there were no graves in Egypt that you brought us to the desert to die? What have you done to us by bringing us out of Egypt?* 12*Didn't we say to you in Egypt, 'Leave us alone; let us serve the Egyptians'? It would have been better for us to serve the Egyptians than to die in the desert!"*

13*Moses answered the people, "Do not be afraid. Stand firm and you will see the deliverance the LORD will bring you today. The Egyptians you see today you will never see again".*

21*Then Moses stretched out his hand over the sea, and all that night the LORD drove the sea back with a strong east wind and turned it into dry land. The waters were divided,* 22*and the Israelites went through the sea on dry ground, with a wall of water on their right and on their left.*

25*He made the wheels of their chariots come off so that they had difficulty driving. And the Egyptians said, "Let's get away from the Israelites! The LORD is fighting for them against Egypt."*

Imagine the scene. The Israelites had escaped from slavery in Egypt through God's mighty deliverance. They had journeyed as far as the Red Sea, and **now they were trapped**. The impassable

25

sea was in front of them and Pharaoh's mighty army behind them. **There was no way out of their terrible situation, and they panicked**.

v 10 *"They were terrified and cried out to the LORD."*

v 12 *"It would have been better for us to serve the Egyptians than to die in the desert."*

Are you in a state of panic like this about your insurmountable and dire, insoluble state of affairs? **Feel your panic**, don't try to push it aside.

v 13 *"Moses answered the people, 'Do not be afraid'. "*

Moses **had faith** in God to surmount the problem. Meditate on the power of God until you have it. Think of all the ways He has proved Himself to help and deliver you in the past.

v 13 *"Stand firm* [or *still*]*"*

There is a time for going to others for help, but when all has failed – stop doing it – **just stand firm on God's promises and His care for you**.

Meditate until you are quiet in your own mind and heart, and your whole being is relaxed. **Wait** for God to fulfil His promises and answer your prayers.

v 13 *"you will see the deliverance the LORD will bring you today. 14The LORD will fight for you; you need only to be still."*

Meditate until you believe that this promise is for you **personally**.

v 22 *"the Israelites went through the sea on dry ground"*

The unthinkable, the impossible happened – they went through their problems to the other side. This will be the result of God's action for you.

Meditate until **you** are also sure, and return to this meditation until you have come through your problem and have left it behind.

Personal notes

A MEDITATION FOR THOSE WHO ARE SICK, PHYSICALLY OR MENTALLY

This is one of the most wonderful revelations of God's nature and purposes in the whole Bible.

Exodus 15 verses 25b-26

25b *"There the LORD made a decree and a law for them, and there He tested them.*

26*He said, 'If you listen carefully to the voice of the LORD your God and do what is right in his eyes, if you pay attention to his commands and keep all his decrees, I will not bring on you any of the diseases I brought on the Egyptians, for I am the LORD, who heals you'."*

Meditation: 'I AM' is the name of God (YAHWEH or

JEHOVAH). It reveals not only His name but His **nature**.

1   Meditate on all you know or have experienced about God's blessings upon your life and all that this reveals to you about God – His love, His power, His will, not only for you but for all His children.

2   *"the LORD"*
Meditate on the sovereignty of God – His omnipotent rule over all nature and mankind, and His ultimate ability to bring to pass all that He promises.

3   *"who heals you"*
Meditate on what His will is for you; your body, and your mind. The Hebrew words can be translated, "I am the Lord your physician". His Name, His nature and His absolute promise is to **heal you**.

4   Imagine, feel and experience God's healing power flowing through the depths of your mind and also your body from your head to your toes. Meditate on God; draw near to God; pray to Him; open all your being to Him in deep communion with Him and keep this verse of Scripture **always** before you and in your heart.

Personal notes

A MEDITATION FOR THOSE WHO ARE AFRAID, SPIRITUALLY DISHEARTENED OR SPIRITUALLY DEPRESSED

Read I Kings 18 v 16-end.
Passage for meditation:
I Kings 19 verses 1-18

1*Now Ahab told Jezebel everything Elijah had done and how he had killed all the prophets with the sword.* 2*So Jezebel sent a messenger to Elijah to say, "May the gods deal with me, be it ever so severely if by this time tomorrow I do not make your life like that of one of them."*

3*Elijah was afraid and ran for his life. When he came to Beersheba in Judah, he left his servant there,* 4*while he himself went a day's journey into the desert. He came to a broom tree, sat down under it and prayed that he might die. "I have had enough, LORD," he said. "Take my life, I am no better than my ancestors."* 5*Then he lay down under the tree and fell asleep.*

All at once an angel touched him and said, "Get up and eat." 6*He looked around, and there by his head was a cake of bread baked over hot coals, and a jar of water. He ate and drank and then lay down again.*

7*The angel of the LORD came back a second time and said, "Get up and eat, for the journey is too much for you."* 8*So he got up and ate and drank. Strengthened by that food, he travelled for forty days and forty nights until he reached Horeb, the mountain of God.* 9*There he went into a cave and spent the night.*

And the word of the LORD came to him: "What are you doing here, Elijah?"

10He replied, "I have been very zealous for the LORD God Almighty. The Israelites have rejected your covenant, broken down your altars, and put your prophets to death with the sword. I am the only one left, and now they are trying to kill me too."

11The LORD said, "Go out and stand on the mountain in the presence of the LORD, for the LORD is about to pass by."

Then a great and powerful wind tore the mountains apart and shattered the rocks before the LORD, but the LORD was not in the wind. After the wind there was an earthquake, but the LORD was not in the earthquake. 12After the earthquake came a fire, but the LORD was not in the fire. And after the fire came a gentle whisper. 13When Elijah heard it, he pulled his cloak over his face and went out and stood at the mouth of the cave.

Then a voice said to him, "What are you doing here, Elijah?"

14He replied, "I have been very zealous for the LORD God Almighty. The Israelites have rejected your covenant, broken down your altars, and put your prophets to death with the sword. I am the only one left, and now they are trying to kill me too."

15The LORD said to him, "Go back the way you came, and go to the desert of Damascus. When you get there, anoint Hazael king over Aram. 16Also, anoint Jehu son of Nimshi king over Israel,and anoint Elisha son of Shaphat from Abel Meholah to succeed you as prophet. 17Jehu will put to death any who escape the sword of Hazael, and Elisha will put to death any who escape the sword of Jehu. 18Yet I reserve seven thousand in Israel – all whose knees have not bowed down to Baal and all whose mouths have *not kissed him."*

1   Imagine you are Elijah. You have had such tremendous faith.
    You have won a remarkable victory over the prophets of Baal,
    and even had such faith in God that you have caused Him to
    end a terrible drought, and caused it to rain in torrents.
2   Now you have heard that Queen Jezebel (who worshipped
    Baal) is going to have you slaughtered – feel his terror and run
    for your life.
3   Now sit under the broom tree and enter into such agonising
    depression that you pray that you may die. You feel you've
    had enough and say to the Lord, "Take my life, I am no better
    than my ancestors" – then imagine that you fall asleep.
4   *"All at once an angel touched him and said, 'Get up and
    eat.' He looked around and there by his head was a cake of
    bread baked over hot coals, and a jar of water. He ate and
    drank and then lay down again."*
    Feel the angel's touch and wake up and see the cake of bread
    and jar of water near to you.
5   *"The angel of the LORD came back a second time and
    touched him and said, 'Get up and eat, for the journey is too
    much for you.'   So he got up and ate and drank.
    Strengthened by that food, he travelled for forty days and
    forty nights until he reached Horeb,* [Sinai] *the mountain of
    God. There he went into a cave and spent the night."*
    Hear the angel's voice, and eat and drink – then go on your
    journey to a cave on Mount Horeb, and spend the night there.
6   *"And the word of the LORD came to him, 'What are you
    doing here, Elijah?'*
    *He replied, 'I have been very zealous for the LORD God
    Almighty.   The Israelites have rejected your covenant,*

broken down your altars, and put your prophets to death with the sword. I am the only one left, and now they are trying to kill me too.' "

Hear the voice of the Lord speaking these words to you, and speak your complaint to Him. Then go and stand on the mountain and feel the presence of the Lord.

7　*"Then a great and powerful wind tore the mountains apart and shattered the rocks before the LORD, but the LORD was not in the wind. After the wind there was an earthquake, but the LORD was not in the earthquake. After the earthquake came a fire, but the LORD was not in the fire. And after the fire came a gentle whisper.*
When Elijah heard it, he pulled his cloak over his face and went out and stood at the mouth of the cave.

Then a voice said to him, 'What are you doing here, Elijah?'

He replied, 'I have been very zealous for the LORD God Almighty. The Israelites have rejected your covenant, broken down your altars, and put your prophets to death with the sword. I am the only one left, and now they are trying to kill me too.' "

Hear and feel the powerful wind. Then feel the earth quake under your feet. See and feel the heat of the fire. Then hear the gentle whisper. Then once again describe to God what you see as your terrible plight.

8　*"The LORD said to him, 'Go back the way you came, and go to the desert of Damascus. When you get there, anoint Hazael king over Aram. Also, anoint Jehu son of Nimshi king over Israel, and anoint Elisha son of Shaphat from Abel Meholah to succeed you as prophet. Jehu will put to death any who escape the sword of Hazael, and Elisha will put to*

death any who escape the sword of Jehu.
Yet I reserve seven thousand in Israel – all whose knees have not bowed down to Baal and all whose mouths have not kissed him.' "

Hear the Lord's command and what He knows of the spiritual situation in Israel.

a) See how often spiritual depression can follow wonderful spiritual experiences, real faith, and demonstrations of God's power.

b) See how fear and *self-pity* are devastating emotions which can bring you into deep depression.

c) See how God actually knows your condition and sympathises with it. Hear the words: "What are you doing here?" – in this woeful condition and lack of trust in God.

d) See how God is with you in your depression and has made provision for you to come out of it.

e) Feel His strength and upliftment come into your mind.

f) Hear Him speak to you, not in dramatic ways or events but in a gentle whisper.

g) See that He still has work for you to do for Him, and get up and do it.

Personal notes

MEDITATION (2) FOR THOSE WHO ARE PHYSICALLY OR EMOTIONALLY SICK

2 Kings 5 verses 1-14

1Now Naaman was commander of the army of the king of Aram. He was a great man in the sight of his master and highly regarded, because through him the LORD had given victory to Aram. He was a valiant soldier, but he had leprosy.

2Now bands from Aram had gone out and had taken captive a young girl from Israel, and she served Naaman's wife. 3She said to her mistress, "If only my master would see the prophet who is in Samaria! He would cure him of his leprosy."

4Naaman went to his master and told him what the girl from Israel had said. 5"By all means, go," the king of Aram said. "I will send a letter to the king of Israel." So Naaman left, taking with him ten talents of silver, six thousand shekels of gold and ten sets of clothing. 6The letter that he took to the king of Israel read, "With this letter I am sending my servant Naaman to you so that you may cure him of his leprosy."

7As soon as the king of Israel read the letter, he tore his robes and said, "Am I God? Can I kill and bring back to life?

Why does this fellow send someone to me to be cured of his leprosy? See how he is trying to pick a quarrel with me!"

8When Elisha thr man of God heard that the king of Israel had torn his robes, he sent him this message: "Why have you torn your robes? Make the man come to me and he will know that there is a prophet in Israel." 9So Naaman went with his horses and chariots and stopped at the door of Elisha's house. 10Elisha sent a messenger to say to him, "Go, wash yourself seven times in the Jordan, and your flesh will be restored and you will be cleansed."

11But Naaman went away angry and said, "I thought that he would surely come out to me and stand and call on the name of the LORD his God, wave his hand over the spot and cure me of my leprosy. 12Are not Abana and Pharpar, the rivers of Damascus, better than any of the waters of Israel? Couldn't I wash in them and be cleansed?" So he turned and went off in a rage.

13Naaman's servants went to him and said, "My father, if the prophet had told you to do some great thing, would you not have done it? How much more, then, when he tells you, 'Wash and be cleansed'?" 14So he went down and dipped himself in the Jordan seven times, as the man of God had told him, and his flesh was restored and became clean like that of a young boy.

1   Imagine you are Naaman: a great man, powerful, physically basically strong, rich, popular, a valiant soldier, every mother's dream of what her son might become. However, there is a terrible 'but' in your life, a dreadful impediment – you have leprosy. This means that in time – 'terminal'.

2   Then a young girl, a slave girl, the lowest of the low in your

household, has said something remarkable to your wife, who has passed it on to you – *"She said to her mistress, 'If only my master would see the prophet who is in Samaria! He would cure him of his leprosy'."*

3   You go to the King who gives you permission to go to this prophet of whom you have never heard and is in a foreign, even hostile country. So you go; but you are a proud man; you will pay for your healing with material wealth – *" 'By all means, go,' the king of Aram replied. 'I will send a letter to the king of Israel.' So Naaman left, taking with him ten talents of silver, six thousand shekels of gold and ten sets of clothing. The letter that he took to the king of Israel read: 'With this letter I am sending my servant Naaman to you so that you may cure him of his leprosy'."*

4   You take the letter to the king of Israel, who is absolutely faithless that any such miracle can take place – *"As soon as the king of Israel read the letter, he tore his robes and said, 'Am I God? Can I kill and bring back to life? Why does this fellow send someone to me to be cured of his leprosy? See how he is trying to pick a quarrel with me!'*

5   Elisha the prophet hears about all this and says that by God's power the miracle will be effected, and so you go to the prophet's small dwelling.

6   The prophet doesn't even bother to come out to see you, but sends a messenger with a strange command – *"Elisha sent a messenger to say to him, 'Go, wash yourself seven times in the Jordan, and your flesh will be restored and you will be cleansed'."*

7   You become very angry and say: *" 'I thought that he would surely come out to me and stand and call on the name of*

the LORD his God, wave his hand over the spot and cure me of my leprosy.   Are not Abana and Pharpar, the rivers of Damascus, better than any of the waters of Israel? Couldn't I wash in them and be cleansed?' "

8   Your servants persuade you to obey the prophet and you decide to do so – *"So he went down and dipped himself in the Jordan seven times, as the man of God had told him, and his flesh was restored and became clean like that of a young boy."*

Meditate on:
1   whatever sickness or 'but' you have in your life which seems hopeless.
2   the bold and absolutely trusting way we must testify to the power of God.
3   God's absolute power to work a miracle for you.
4   the importance of obedience to God, however strange His commands may seem.
5   the fact that it is faith, not wealth, or work, that will bring the miracle to pass.

Personal notes

A MEDITATION FOR THOSE WHO ARE FEARFUL ABOUT WORLD AFFAIRS

Psalm 2

1*Why do the nations conspire*
and the peoples plot in vain?
2*The kings of the earth take their stand*
and the rulers gather together against the LORD
and against his Anointed One.
3*"Let us break their chains," they say,*
"and throw off their fetters."

4*The One enthroned in heaven laughs;*
the Lord scoffs at them.
5*Then he rebukes them in his anger*
and terrifies them in his wrath, saying,
6*"I have installed my King*
on Zion, my holy hill."

7*I will proclaim the decree of the LORD:*

He said to me, "You are my Son;
today I have become your Father.
8*Ask of me, and I will make the nations your inheritance,*
the ends of the earth your possession.
9*You will rule them with an iron sceptre;*
you will dash them to pieces like pottery."
10*Therefore, you kings, be wise;*
be warned, you rulers of the earth.
11*Serve the LORD with fear*
and rejoice with trembling.
12*Kiss the Son, lest he be angry*
and you be destroyed in your way,
for his wrath can flare up in a moment.
Blessed are all who take refuge in him.

This is a 'Messianic' psalm, because it is all about Jesus.

"Why do the nations conspire and the peoples plot in vain? The kings of the earth take their stand and the rulers gather together against the LORD and against his Anointed One. 'Let us break their chains,' they say, 'and throw off their fetters.'
Meditate on the ways in which peoples and nations have rejected God and Jesus, "His anointed One". They have rebelled against God and have rebelled against His rule over them – this is the fundamental reason why there is so much conflict and evil.

"The One enthroned in heaven laughs; the Lord scoffs at them. Then he rebukes them in his anger and terrifies them in his wrath, saying, 'I have installed my King on Zion, my holy hill'."

Meditate on God's view of all this and His absolute sovereignty – He is not threatened nor is His throne under siege.

V. 5 speaks again of Jesus. Meditate on His Ascension to rule on high.

"I will proclaim the decree of the LORD:
He said to me, 'You are my Son; today I have become your Father. Ask of me, and I will make the nations your inheritance, the ends of the earth your possession'."
Meditate again on the place of Jesus in the eventual dominion and how the world will end.

" 'You will rule them with an iron sceptre; you will dash them to pieces like pottery.' Therefore, you kings, be wise; be warned, you rulers of the earth. Serve the LORD with fear and rejoice with trembling."
Meditate – in the light of verses 7-9 what ought the nations to do?

"Kiss the Son, lest he be angry and you be destroyed in your way, for his wrath can flare up in a moment. Blessed are all who take refuge in him."
Meditate on the wrath of God – His righteous indignation against evil in the world.

Personal notes

A MEDITATION ON
PRAISING THE LORD

Psalm 9

1I will praise You, O LORD, with all my heart;
I will tell of all Your wonders.
2I will be glad and rejoice in You;
I will sing praise to Your name, O Most High.

3My enemies turn back;
they stumble and perish before You.
4For You have upheld my right and my cause;
You have sat on Your throne, judging righteously.
5You have rebuked the nations and destroyed the wicked;
You have blotted out their name for ever and ever.
6Endless ruin has overtaken the enemy,
You have uprooted their cities;
even the memory of them has perished.

7The LORD reigns for ever;
He has established His throne for judgment.
8He will judge the world in rughteousness;

He will govern the peoples with justice.
9The LORD is a refuge for the oppressed,
a stronghold in times of trouble.
10Those who know Your name will trust in You,
for You, O LORD, have never forsaken those who seek You.

11Sing praises to the LORD, enthroned in Zion;
proclaim among the nations what He has done.
12For He who avenges blood remembers;
He does not ignore the cry of the afflicted.

13O LORD, see how my enemies persecute me!
Have mercy and lift me up from the gates of death,
14that I may declare Your praises
in the gates of the Daughter of Zion
and there rejoice in Your salvation.
15The nations have fallen into the pit they have dug;
their feet are caught in the net they have hidden.
16The LORD is known by His justice;
the wicked are ensnared by the work of their hands.

17The wicked return to the grave,
all the nations that forget God.
18But the needy will not always be forgotten,
nor the hope of the afflicted ever perish.

19Arise, O LORD, let not man triumph;
let the nations be judged in Your presence.
20Strike them with terror, O LORD;
let the nations know they are but men.

v 1 *"I will praise You, O LORD, with all my heart*
I will tell of all Your wonders".

Meditation: What does it mean to praise the Lord **with all my heart**? This comes from meditating on all **His wonders** – meditate on all He has done for mankind, especially in Jesus – meditate on all He has done for you.

v 2 *"I will be glad and rejoice in You;*
I will sing praise to Your name, O Most High."

With the psalmist rejoice and be glad in Him – in who He is in himself – and literally sing praises to Him the best way you can – in tongues if you have that gift.

vv3-6 *"My enemies turn back; they stumble and perish before You. For You have upheld my right and my cause; You have sat on Your throne, judging righteously.*
You have rebuked the nations and destroyed the wicked; You have blotted out their name for ever and ever.
Endless ruin has overtaken the enemy, You have uprooted their cities; even the memory of them has perished."

We Christians' enemies are Satan and all his army of spiritual and mortal evildoers – praise God for His victory over them in Jesus' death, resurrection and ascension – meditate on how He has delivered you and what it means to live the victorious life.

vv 7-8 *"The LORD reigns for ever; He has established His throne for judgment.*
He will judge the world in righteousness; He will govern the peoples with justice."

The Lord reigns – meditate on the fact that nothing is outside His eventual control over all things on earth and in your life.

vv 9-10 *"The LORD is a refuge for the oppressed, a stronghold in times of trouble.*

Those who know Your name will trust in You, for You, LORD, have never forsaken those who seek You."

Meditate on the Lord being a **refuge** and **stronghold** – and consequently on the trust you can put in Him.

Meditate on the promise: "for You, Lord, have **never** forsaken those who seek You".

v 11 *"Sing praises to the LORD, enthroned in Zion; proclaim among the nations what He has done."*

His praise must resound not only from your lips, but also among the nations – meditate on the worldwide people of God who at all times are praising Him – join with them.

vv 13-16 *"O LORD, see how my enemies persecute me! Have mercy and lift me up from the gates of death, that I may declare Your praises in the gates of the Daughter of Zion and there rejoice in Your salvation.*

The nations have fallen into the pit they have dug; their feet are caught in the net they have hidden.

The LORD is known by His justice; the wicked are ensnared by the work of their hands."

Meditate on the fact that you should praise Him even when things are going wrong for you and you feel 'down'.

vv 17-19 *"The wicked return to the grave, all the nations that forget God. But the needy will not always be forgotten, nor the hope of the afflicted ever perish.*

Arise, O LORD, let not man triumph, let the nations be

judged in Your presence."

Praise God that He will always triumph in the world and in your life.

Personal notes

A MEDITATION FOR THOSE WHO ARE DEPRESSED

Sufferers from depression are obviously not happy. They have an illness affecting the emotional aspect of their life. They certainly lack any kind of joy. The following psalm indicates a spiritual way to find deep joy, especially as a sufferer from this illness repeatedly and deeply meditates upon it.

Psalm 16

1Keep me safe, O God,
for in You I find refuge.

2I said to the LORD, "You are my Lord;
apart from You I have no good thing."
3As for the saints who are in the land,
they are the glorious ones
in whom is all my delight.
4The sorrows of those will increase
who run after other gods.
I will not pour out their libations of blood
or take up their names on my lips.

5LORD, You have assigned me my portion and my cup;
You have made my lot secure.
6The boundary lines have fallen for me
in pleasant places;
surely I have a delightful inheritance.

7I will praise the LORD, who counsels me;
even at night my heart instructs me.
8I have set the LORD always before me.
Because He is at my right hand,
I shall not be shaken.

9Therefore my heart is glad and my tongue rejoices;
my body also will rest secure,
10because You will not abandon me to the grave,
nor will You let Your Holy One see decay.
11You have made known to me the path of life;
You will fill me with joy in Your presence,
with eternal pleasures at Your right hand.

1.   v 1 *"Keep me safe, O God, for in You I take refuge."*
Meditate on the profound security that can be found in God
alone.

2.   v 2 *"I said to the LORD, 'You are my Lord; apart from You
I have no good thing'."*
Meditate on the fact that the answer to your problem rests in
God **alone**.

3.   v 3 *"As for the saints who are in the land, they are the
glorious ones in whom is all my delight."*
Meditate on the **delight** which can be found in prayer, worship
and the fellowship of God's people — those who really know
Him and communicate spiritual truths.

4. v 4 *"The sorrows of those will increase who run after other gods."*
Meditate on whether you are seeking and desiring – yearning for anything or anybody other than **God alone**.

5. v 5 *"LORD, You have assigned me my portion and my cup; You have made my lot secure."*
Meditate until you are fully satisfied with all in your life situation as it has been appointed by God and therefore is secure.

6. v 6 *"The boundary lines have fallen for me in pleasant places; surely I have a delightful inheritance."*
Meditate on all the good things – the blessings you have in your life – and thank God for them **from your heart**.

7. v 7 *"I will praise the LORD, who counsels me; even at night my heart instructs me."*
Meditate on the Lord, who really is your best counsellor. Spend time listening to His counsel even during sleepless nights.

8. v 9 *"Therefore my heart is glad and my tongue rejoices; my body also will rest secure"*
Meditate on why this is true: – because (v 8) "I have set the LORD always before me. Because He is at my right hand [giving strength] I shall not be shaken" (nothing can disturb me).

9. v 11 *"You have made known to me the path of life; You will fill me with joy in Your presence,*

with eternal pleasures at Your right hand."
Meditate on the fact that God has guided your life right up to this moment and will do so in the future. In Him alone – His presence with you every hour of day and night – even in your depression – when you can't feel His nearness He will, if you ask Him, fill you with the joy which comes from Himself, and you will, as you delight in **Him** – not yourself – not focusing on cares or worries of this life – find **eternal** pleasure.

Personal notes

A MEDITATION ON OUR RESPONSE TO GOD REVEALED IN NATURE AND THE LAW

Psalm 19

1The heavens declare the glory of God;
the skies proclaim the work of His hands.
2Day after day they pour forth speech;
night after night they display knowledge.
3There is no speech or language where their voice is not heard.
4Their voice goes out into all the earth,
their words to the ends of the world.

In the heavens He has pitched a tent for the sun,
5which is like a bridegroom coming forth from his pavilion,
like a champion rejoicing to run his course.
6It rises at one end of the heavens
and makes its circuit to the other;
nothing is hidden from its heat.

7The law of the LORD is perfect,
reviving the soul.
The statutes of the LORD are trustworthy,
making wise the simple.
8The precepts of the LORD are right,
giving joy to the heart.
The commands of the LORD are radiant,
giving light to the eyes.

9The fear of the LORD is pure,
enduring for ever.
The ordinances of the LORD are sure
and altogether righteous.
10They are more precious than gold,
than much pure gold;
they are sweeter than honey,
than honey from the comb.
11By them is Your servant warned;
in keeping them there is great reward.

12Who can discern his errors?
Forgive my hidden faults.
13Keep Your servant also from wilful sins;
may they not rule over me.
Then will I be blameless,
innocent of great transgression.

14May the words of my mouth
and the meditation of my heart
be pleasing in Your sight,
O LORD, my Rock and my Redeemer.

v 1 *"The heavens declare the glory of God; the skies
proclaim the work of His hands."*
Meditate on the way the heavens and skies reveal the majesty and
the wonder of God.

v 2 *"Day after day they pour forth speech; night after night
they display knowledge."*
Meditate on the glory of God being revealed worldwide.

vv 4b,5 *"In the heavens He has pitched a tent for the sun, which is like a bridegroom coming forth from his pavilion, like a champion rejoicing to run his course."*
Meditate on the sun and the way it reveals God materially and spiritually.

v 7 *"The law of the LORD is perfect, reviving the soul. The statutes of the LORD are trustworthy, making wise the simple."*
Meditate on how the written word – the whole Bible – reveals the nature of God to you – it is trustworthy and makes the simple wise – meditate on the wisdom it brings to you.

vv 8-10 *"The precepts of the LORD are right, giving joy to the heart. The commands of the LORD are radiant, giving light to the eyes. The fear of the LORD is pure, enduring for ever. The ordinances of the LORD are sure and altogether righteous. They are more precious than gold, than much pure gold; they are sweeter than honey, than honey from the comb."*
Meditate on the way the Bible's truths bring joy to the heart and give light to your life; that they will never pass away – that they are **sure**, more precious than gold and sweeter than honey.

v 11 *"By them is Your servant warned; in keeping them there is great reward."*
Meditate on the way the precepts of the Lord guide us through our lives and so bring their own rewards in happiness and contentment.

vv 12-13 *"Who can discern his errors? Forgive my hidden*

faults. Keep Your servant also from wilful sins; may they not rule over me. Then will I be blameless, innocent of great transgression."

Ask God to forgive all your sins, especially those deep in your heart, and ask God to keep you from wilful sins.

v 14   *"May the words of my mouth and the meditation of my heart be pleasing in Your sight, O LORD, my Rock and my Redeemer."*

Meditate on the use of the words of your mouth, and ask that the deep reflective thoughts that go through your mind will always be pleasing to God, who is a **Rock** and a **Redeemer**.

Personal notes

PSALM 23

The Lord is my shepherd, I shall not be in want..
He makes me lie down in green pastures,
He leads me beside quiet waters, He restores my soul.
He guides me in paths of righteousness for His name's sake.
Even though I walk through the valley of the shadow of death,
I will fear no evil, for You are with me;
Your rod and Your staff they comfort me.
You prepare a table before me in the presence of my enemies.
You anoint my head with oil; my cup overflows.
Surely goodness and love will follow me all the days of my life,
And I will dwell in the house of the LORD for ever.

Read the psalm through at least twice each day and imagine yourself in a lovely, warm, sunny day on the hill slopes of Galilee like David, sitting on the hillside watching over his flock of sheep, and, at the same time thinking deeply about God and likening his relationship with Him to his own with his sheep.

DAY ONE: reflect on the words *"the Lord is my shepherd"*.
This speaks of RELATIONSHIP WITH GOD.
Meditate on your own relationship with Him — e.g. how it came about, what it means to you and what it entails.
God took the initiative in this relationship — THANK HIM.

DAY TWO: *"I shall not be in want"*
Meditate on how God has supplied all your needs.
Think of each one specifically, and how you can trust Him to supply all your needs. THANK HIM.

DAY THREE: *"He makes me lie down in green pastures"*
This speaks of REST: Meditate on times when God has given you
needed rest in body, mind and spirit.
Relax and rest in Him now. Really rest – THANK HIM.

DAY FOUR: *"He leads me beside quiet waters"*
This speaks of REFRESHMENT.
Meditate on times when God has refreshed you. How has He
done it? Again how He refreshes you in body, mind and spirit.
Do you need this refreshment now? Seek it. Feel it. THANK HIM.

DAY FIVE: *"He restores my soul."*
This speaks of RESTORATION, of HEALING – again in body,
mind and spirit – are there places or spheres of your life, e.g. love,
marriage, communion with Him, your whole spiritual life, your
body which need restoration/healing? Seek it. Feel it.
THANK HIM.

DAY SIX *"He guides me in paths of righteousness"*
Meditate on God's promise to guide His people. Trace how He
has guided your life in the past. Do you need His guidance now?
Ask Him. Trust Him. Thank Him.

DAY SEVEN *"For His name's sake."*
Meditate on all that God's/Jesus' Name means to you, and on all
that God has promised in revealing His Name, especially His
Name of Jesus. This text speaks of PURPOSE – to live to glorify
His Name in our daily lives.
What is God's purpose for you? Thank Him that you have a real
purpose in living.

DAY EIGHT   *"Even though I walk through the valley of the shadow of death"*
This speaks of **testing**. Meditate on the reason why God tests you and any tests of faith you have been through or are going through and even meditate on death for a Christian. THANK HIM that He has brought you through.

DAY NINE *"I will fear no evil"*
This speaks of PROTECTION. Meditate ruthlessly on all your fears and on God's present and past protection — you are still alive! Thank Him that He is protecting you.

DAY TEN. *"For You are with me"*
This speaks of FAITHFULNESS. Meditate on "Great is Thy faithfulness, O God my Father" — and on His past faithfulness to you. Thank Him that He is always faithful — never changing.

DAY ELEVEN. *"Your rod and your staff, they comfort me."*
Meditate on the comfort you can find in God. Nothing can separate you from His love (Romans 8). Do you need comforting? Wait on God's comfort — feel it and thank Him for it.

DAY TWELVE. *"You prepare a table before me in the presence of my enemies."*
This speaks of HOPE in all circumstances of your life. Have you lost hope in any way? "Put your hope in God" (Psalm 42 v 5). Meditate on this. Thank Him that there is no hopeless situation in Him.

DAY THIRTEEN. *"You anoint my head with oil"*
This, in the Bible, means consecration. Meditate on what it means

to be consecrated to God. Do you need now to make an act of will to be totally consecrated to God? Thank Him that He will accept your life totally given to Him.

DAY FOURTEEN. *"My cup overflows."*
God's **abundant** blessings. Meditate on His blessings to you. Thank Him for them.

DAY FIFTEEN. *"Surely goodness and love will follow me all the days of my life"*
What a promise of **blessing!** Meditate on what it means to you and thank Him for His promises.

DAY SIXTEEN. *"And I will dwell in the house of the LORD for ever."*
What security! Meditate on eternity and eternal life which He has promised you! Thank Him for it.

Personal notes

A MEDITATION FOR TRUST IN TROUBLE

Psalm 27

1The LORD is my light and my salvation –
whom shall I fear?
The LORD is the stronghold of my life –
of whom shall I be afraid?
2When evil men advance against me
to devour my flesh,
when my enemies and my foes attack me,
they will stumble and fall.
3Though an army besiege me,
my heart will not fear;
though war break out against me,
even then will I be confident.

4One thing I ask of the LORD, this is what I seek:
that I may dwell in the house of the LORD
all the days of my life,
to gaze upon the beauty of the LORD
and to seek Him in His temple.
5For in the day of trouble
He will keep me safe in His dwelling;
He will hide me in the shelter of His tabernacle
and set me high upon a rock.
6Then my head will be exalted
above the enemies who surround me;

at His tabernacle will I sacrifice with shouts of joy;
    I will sing and make music to the LORD.

    7Hear my voice when I call, O LORD;
    be merciful to me and answer me.
    8My heart says of You, "Seek His face!"
    Your face, LORD, I will seek.
    9Do not hide Your face from me,
    do not turn Your servant away in anger;
    You have been my helper.
    Do not reject me or forsake me,
    O God my Saviour.
    10Though my father and mother forsake me,
    the LORD will receive me.
    11Teach me Your way, O LORD;
lead me in a straight path because of my oppressors.
    12Do not hand me over to the desire of my foes,
    for false witnesses rise up against me,
    breathing out violence.

    13I am still confident of this:
    I will see the goodness of the LORD
    in the land of the living.
    14Wait for the LORD;
    be strong and take heart
    and wait for the LORD.

v 1 *"The LORD is my light and my salvation – whom shall I fear? The LORD is the stronghold of my life – of whom shall I be afraid?"*
Meditation – unshakable trust in God.

v 2-3 *"When evil men advance against me to devour my flesh, when my enemies and my foes attack me, they stumble and fall. Though an army besiege me, my heart will not fear; though war break out against me, even then will I be confident."*

Meditation – no matter what trouble you are in – no matter how absolutely terrible the troubles are that assail you – God is on your side and will overcome them.

v 4 *"One thing I ask of the LORD, this is what I seek: that I may dwell in the house of the LORD all the days of my life, to gaze upon the beauty of the LORD and to seek Him in His temple."*

Meditate on your constant relationship with God.

vv 5-6a *"For in the day of trouble He will keep me safe in His dwelling; He will hide me in the shelter of His tabernacle and set me high upon a rock. Then my head will be exalted above the enemies who surround me;"*

Meditate on God's protection and His vindication of you in the end.

v 6b *"at His tabernacle will I sacrifice with shouts of joy; I will sing and make music to the LORD."*

Meditation – on praising God despite and through your troubles and the certainty that you will praise Him for your deliverance.

vv 7-12 *"Hear my voice when I call, O LORD, be merciful to me and answer me. My heart says of You, 'Seek His face!' Your face, LORD, I will seek. Do not hide Your face from me, do not turn Your servant away in anger; You have been my*

helper. Do not reject me or forsake me, O God my Saviour. Though my father and mother forsake me, the LORD will receive me. Teach me Your way, O LORD; lead me in a straight path because of my oppressors. Do not hand me over to the desire of my foes, for false witnesses rise up against me, breathing out violence."
Make this your prayer and meditate upon what it says, and upon God's acceptance of you.

v 13   *"I am still confident of this: I will see the goodness of the LORD in the land of the living."*
Meditate on the trust and patience you need at this time and the way God will strengthen you through it.

Personal notes

A MEDITATION FOR THOSE WHO HAVE LOST HOPE

Introduction: The Babylonians had swept through the land of the Israelites, conquering all that lay before them. The psalmist had witnessed all this but was sure Yahweh would intervene and not allow Jerusalem and especially the Temple to be trodden underfoot. However, the worst imaginable catastrophe had happened and now his hope had gone. Then he sings this lament.

Psalm 42

[1]As the deer pants for streams of water,
　　so my soul pants for You, O God.
[2]My soul thirsts for God, for the living God.
　　When can I go and meet with God?
[3]My tears have been my food day and night,
　　while men say to me all day long,
　　　　"Where is your God?"
[4]These things I remember
　　as I pour out my soul:
how I used to go with the multitude,
leading the procession to the house of God,
　　with shouts of joy and thanksgiving
　　　　among the festive throng.
[5]Why are you downcast, O my soul?
　　Why so disturbed within me?
　　　　Put your hope in God,
　　　　for I will yet praise Him,

my Saviour and my God.
⁶My soul is downcast within me;
therefore I will remember You
from the land of the Jordan,
the heights of Hermon – from Mount Mizar.
⁷Deep calls to deep
in the roar of Your waterfalls;
all Your waves and breakers have swept over me.
⁸By day the LORD directs His love,
at night His song is with me –
a prayer to the God of my life.
⁹I say to God my Rock,
"Why have You forgotten me?
Why must I go about mourning,
oppressed by the enemy?"
¹⁰My bones suffer mortal agony
as my foes taunt me,
saying to me all day long,
"Where is your God?"
¹¹Why are you downcast, O my soul?
Why so disturbed within me?
Put your hope in God,
for I will yet praise Him,
my Saviour and my God.

Psalm 43

¹Vindicate me, O God,
and plead my cause against an ungodly nation;
rescue me from deceitful and wicked men.
²You are God my stronghold.

Why have You rejected me?
Why must I go about mourning,
oppressed by the enemy?
³Send forth Your light and Your truth,
let them guide me;
let them bring me to Your holy mountain,
to the place where You dwell.
⁴Then will I go to the altar of God,
to God, my joy and my delight.
I will praise You with the harp, O God, my God.
⁵Why are you downcast, O my soul?
Why so disturbed within me?
Put your hope in God,
for I will yet praise Him,
my Saviour and my God.

1   vv 1-2 *"As the deer pants for streams of water, so my soul pants for You, O God. My soul thirsts for God, for the living God. When can I go and meet with God?"* Meditation: what does it feel like to '**pant** for God' like a thirsty deer panting for the streams of water? Imagine it. What does it mean to **thirst** for God? Thirst for Him – the living God, and really meet with Him in your meditation.

2   v 3 *"My tears have been my food day and night, while men say to me all day long, 'Where is your God?' "* Meditation: feel this man's despair. Meditate and feel your own despair. Where is God in your salvation?

3   v 4 *"These things I remember as I pour out my soul: how I used to go with the multitude, leading the*

procession to the house of God, with shouts of joy and thanksgiving among the festive throng."
Meditate on all God's past blessings to you in your life.

4   v 5   *"Why are you downcast, O my soul? Why so disturbed within me? Put your hope in God, for I will yet praise Him, my Saviour and my God."*
Meditation – in view of (3) verse 4, renew your hope in God. Meditate until your hope is restored.

5   v 7   *"Deep calls to deep in the roar of Your waterfalls; all Your waves and breakers have swept over me."*
Meditate on what it means for the deepest parts of your inner being to meet at depth with the innermost being of God.

6   v 8   *"By day the LORD directs His love, at night His song is with me – a prayer to the God of my life."*
Meditate on the love of God and what it means to sing to the 'God of your life'.

7   vv 9-11   *"I say to God my Rock, 'Why have You forgotten me? Why must I go about mourning, oppressed by the enemy?' My bones suffer mortal agony as my foes taunt me, saying to me all day long, 'Where is your God?' Why are you downcast, O my soul? Why so disturbed within me?   Put your hope in God, for I will yet praise Him, my Saviour and my God."*
Meditation: again feel the despair, and once again put your hope in God – and believe with the psalmist that absolutely certainly your God will answer your need and you will again

praise your Saviour and your God.

8 **Psalm 43** v 2   *"You are God my stronghold. Why have You rejected me? Why must I go about mourning, oppressed by the enemy?"*
   Meditate: what does it mean to have God as your 'stronghold'?

9 v 3 *"Send forth Your light and Your truth, let them guide me; let them bring me to Your holy mountain, to the place where You dwell."*
   Pray this with the psalmist and enter into what it means.

10 v 4 *"Then will I go to the altar of God, to God, my joy and my delight. I will praise You with the harp, O God, my God."*
   Meditate − this is the certain result of your faith in God − **praise Him aloud**.

11 v 5 *"Why are you downcast, O my soul? Why so disturbed within me? Put your hope in God, for I will yet praise Him, my Saviour and my God."*
   Meditate on this **certainty** and share the psalmist's faith in a wonderful outcome to your need.

Personal notes

A MEDITATION FOR THOSE WHO FEEL INSECURE

The security of one who trusts in the Lord

Security is the most important basic human need, especially in the insecure days in which we live.

Psalm 91

[1]He who dwells in the shelter of the Most High
will rest in the shadow of the Almighty.
[2]I will say of the LORD, "He is my refuge
and my fortress, my God, in whom I trust."
[3]Surely He will save you from the fowler's snare
and from the deadly pestilence.
[4]He will cover you with His feathers,
and under His wings you will find refuge;
His faithfulness will be your shield and rampart.
[5]You will not fear the terror of night,
nor the arrow that flies by day,
[6]nor the pestilence that stalks in the darkness,
nor the plague that destroys at midday.
[7]A thousand may fall at your side,

ten thousand at your right hand,
but it will not come near you.
[8]You will only observe with your eyes
and see the punishment of the wicked.

[9]If you make the Most High your dwelling –
even the LORD, who is my refuge –
[10]then no harm will befall you,
no disaster will come near your tent.
[11]For He will command His angels concerning you
to guard you in all your ways;
[12]they will lift you up in their hands,
so that you will not strike your foot against a stone.
[13]You will tread upon the lion and the cobra;
you will trample the great lion and the serpent.
[14]"Because he loves Me," says the LORD, "I will rescue him;
I will protect him, for he acknowledges My name.
[15]He will call upon Me, and I will answer him;
I will be with him in trouble,
I will deliver him and honour him.
[16]With long life will I satisfy him
and show him my salvation."

1   v 1-2   *"He who dwells in the shelter of the Most High
will rest in the shadow of the Almighty.   I will say of the
LORD, 'He is my refuge and my fortress, my God, in
whom I trust'."*
Meditation: 'Most High' speaks of the sovereignty of God –
meditate on the words 'shelter', 'rest', 'refuge', 'fortress'.
God is like a castle – the most formidable place to be in the
world of the psalmist.

2   v 3 *"Surely He will save you from the fowler's snare and from the deadly pestilence."*

3   vv 4-6 *"He will cover you with His feathers, and under His wings you will find refuge; His faithfulness will be your shield and rampart. You will not fear the terror of night, nor the arrow that flies by day, nor the pestilence that stalks in the darkness, nor the plague that destroys at midday."*

God is now declared to be all-powerful in guarding us.

4   vv 7-8 *"A thousand may fall at your side, ten thousand at your right hand, but it will not come near you. You will only observe with your eyes and see the punishment of the wicked."*

Meditate – how no matter if even a thousand people will fall under attack – **you will not**.

5   vv 9-10 *"If you make the Most High your dwelling – even the LORD, who is my refuge – then no harm will befall you, no disaster will come near your tent."*

Meditate on the unshakable promises to you from God Himself – nothing will invade even your home.

6   vv 11-13 *"For He will command His angels concerning you to guard you in all your ways; they will lift you up in their hands, so that you will not strike your foot against a stone. You will tread upon the lion and the cobra; you will trample the great lion and the serpent."*

Meditate on the ministry of angels protecting you, carrying you along a rock-strewn road in the desert.

7   Verses 14-16   *" 'Because he loves Me,' says the LORD, I will rescue him; I will protect him, for he acknowledges My name. He will call upon Me, and I will answer him; I will be with him in trouble, I will deliver him and honour . him. With long life will I satisfy him and show him My salvation'."*

Now God actually speaks to you – meditate on the promises He makes to those who love Him.

Closing thought:

For I am convinced that neither death nor life,
neither angels nor demons,
neither the present nor the future,
nor any powers, neither height nor depth,
nor anything else in all creation,
will be able to separate us from the love of God
that is in Christ Jesus our Lord.

(Romans 8: 38-39)

Personal notes

A MEDITATION ON THANKFULNESS TO GOD FOR HEALING AND FORGIVENESS

Psalm 103

[1]Praise the LORD, O my soul;
all my inmost being, praise His holy name.
[2]Praise the LORD, O my soul,
and forget not all His benefits –
[3]who forgives all your sins and heals all your diseases,
[4]who redeems your life from the pit
and crowns you with love and compassion,
[5]who satisfies your desires with good things
so that your youth is renewed like the eagle's.
[6]The LORD works righteousness and justice for all the oppressed.
[7]He made known His ways to Moses,
His deeds to the people of Israel:
[8]The LORD is compassionate and gracious,
slow to anger, abounding in love.
[9]He will not always accuse,
nor will He harbour His anger for ever;
[10]He does not treat us as our sins deserve
or repay us according to our iniquities.

¹¹For as high as the heavens are above the earth,
so great is His love for those who fear Him;
¹²as far as the east is from the west,
so far has He removed our
transgressions from us.
¹³As a father has compassion on his children,
so the LORD has compassion on those who fear Him;
¹⁴for He knows how we are formed,
He remembers that we ire dust.
¹⁵As for man, his days are like grass,
he flourishes like a flower of the field;
¹⁶the wind blows over it and it is gone,
and its place remembers it no more.
¹⁷But from everlasting to everlasting
the LORD's love is with those who fear Him,
and His righteousness with their children's children –
¹⁸with those who keep His covenant
and remember to obey His precepts.
¹⁹The LORD has established His throne in heaven,
and His kingdom rules over all.
²⁰Praise the LORD, you His angels,
you mighty ones who do His bidding,
who obey His word.
²¹Praise the LORD, all His heavenly hosts,
you His servants who do His will.
²²Praise the LORD, all His works
everywhere in His dominion.
Praise the LORD, O my soul.

1   v 1   *"Praise the LORD, O my soul; all my inmost being,
praise His holy name."*

Meditation: David praises God with his **soul** and his **inmost being**.

2   v 2 *"Praise the LORD, O my soul, and forget not all His benefits"*
Meditate on all God's blessing you have and daily experience.

3   v 3 *"who forgives all your sins and heals all your diseases"*
Meditation – this is a promise to you – notice the word **all**.

4   v 4 *"who redeems your life from the pit and crowns you with love and compassion"*
Meditate on the promise of deliverance from death ... also on God's love and compassion which you should always be experiencing in your life.

5   v 5 *"who satisfies your desires with good things so that your youth is renewed like the eagle's."*
Meditate on these promises God gives us and is the source of all good things.

6   v 6 *"The LORD works righteousness and justice for all the oppressed."*
Meditate on the Lord's care for all who have need.

7   vv 7-13 *"He made known His ways to Moses, His deeds to the people of Israel: the LORD is compassionate and gracious, slow to anger, abounding in love. He will not always accuse, nor will He harbour His anger for ever;*

He does not treat us as our sins deserve or repay us according to our iniquities. For as high as the heavens are above the earth, so great is His love for those who fear Him; as far as the east is from the west, so far has He removed our transgressions from us.
As a father has compassion on his children, so the LORD has compassion on those who fear Him."
Meditate at length on all that these words reveal of the innermost being of God in relation to you. His attributes are all love and compassion.

8 vv 14-18 *"for He knows how we are formed, He remembers that we are dust. As for man, his days are like grass, he flourishes like a flower of the field; the wind blows over it and it is gone, and its place remembers it no more. But from everlasting to everlasting the LORD's love is with those who fear Him, and His righteousness with their children's children – with those who keep His covenant and remember to obey His precepts."*
Meditate on the **eternity** of God in contrast to the finitude of man.

9 v 19 *"The LORD has established His throne in heaven, and His kingdom rules over all."*
Meditate on God's sovereign rule over all His creation including humans.

10 vv 20-22 *"Praise the LORD, you His angels, you mighty ones who do His bidding, who obey His word. Praise the*
LORD, all His heavenly hosts, you His servants who do

His will. Praise the LORD, all His works everywhere in His dominion.
Praise the LORD, O my soul."
Simply praise the Lord aloud and with all your being, using the words of David.

Personal notes

A MEDITATION ABOUT SEVERAL TERRIBLE CONDITIONS

Psalm 107 verses 4-32

4Some wandered in desert wastelands,
finding no way to a city where they could settle.
5They were hungry and thirsty, and their lives ebbed away.
6Then they cried out to the LORD in their trouble,
and He delivered them from their distress.
7He led them by a straight way to a city where they could settle.
8Let them give thanks to the LORD for His unfailing love
and His wonderful deeds for men,
9for He satisfies the thirsty and fills the hungry with good things.

10Some sat in darkness and the deepest gloom,
prisoners suffering in iron chains,
11for they had rebelled against the words of God,
and despised the counsel of the Most High.
12So He subjected them to bitter labour;
they stumbled, and there was no one to help.
13Then they cried to the LORD in their trouble,
and He saved them from their distress.
14He brought them out of darkness and the deepest gloom
and broke away their chains.
15Let them give thanks to the LORD for His unfailing love
and His wonderful deeds for men,
16for He breaks down gates of bronze
and cuts through bars of iron.

17Some became fools through their rebellious ways
and suffered affliction because of their iniquities.
18They loathed all food and drew near the gates of death.
19Then they cried to the LORD in their trouble,
and He saved them from their distress.
20He sent forth His word and healed them,
He rescued them from the grave.
21Let them give thanks to the LORD for His unfailing love
and His wonderful deeds for men.
22Let them sacrifice thank-offerings
and tell of His works with songs of joy.

23Others went out on the sea in ships;
they were merchants on the mighty waters.
24They saw the works of the LORD,
His wonderful deeds in the deep.
25For He spoke and stirred up a tempest
that lifted high the waves.
26They mounted up to the heavens and went down to the depths;
in their peril their courage melted away.
27They reeled and staggered like drunken men;
they were at their wits' end.
28Then they cried out to the LORD in their trouble,
and He brought them out of their distress.
29He stilled the storm to a whisper;
the waves of the sea were hushed.
30They were glad when it grew calm,
And He guided them to their desired haven.
31Let them give thanks to the LORD for His unfailing love
and His wonderful deeds for men.
32Let them exalt Him in the assembly of the people
and praise Him in the council of the elders.

1. **Verses 4-9** speak about those who have become lost. Meditate on what it feels like to be lost on a vital journey –
feel the bewilderment, confusion and even panic. Then picture Jesus finding you. He came to "seek and save that which was lost". Feel the joy of being found by Him and being led on the right path. Then give thanks to the Lord v 8.

2. **Verses 10-16** speak of being a prisoner. Feel the darkness and gloom of an underground prison. Feel the chains which are fastened all around your body – you are in pitch darkness and cannot move. Are you in any bondage of body, mind or spirit? Is there anything from which you cannot break free? Jesus delivered many from bondage. Meditate until you feel set free. Then praise Him vv 15-16.

3. **Verses 17-22** speak of being physically ill. Feel your sickness, your discomfort, your pain at its worst. God will speak His Word into this condition. **"I am the Lord who heals you"** (Exodus 15). Meditate on these words deeply and constantly until you can really praise Him v 21-22 – with joy.

4. **Verses 24-32** speak of circumstances and life going terribly wrong, suddenly and unexpectedly – a storm has hit you! Feel its power. Meditate and imagine you are in a boat, in a storm at sea, reeling and staggering on the deck. Then Jesus speaks into the situation: "Peace, be still!" calming the storm to a whisper. Then praise Him as you feel tranquillity and peace vv 31-32.

Personal notes

A MEDITATION FOR THOSE IN CHRISTIAN SERVICE WHO ARE SUFFERING DISCOURAGEMENT

Psalm 126 verses 4-6

[4]Restore our fortunes,` O LORD,
like streams in the Negev.
[5]Those who sow tears
will reap with songs of joy.
[6]He who goes out weeping,
carrying seed to sow,
will return with songs of joy,
carrying sheaves with him.

I would like you to meditate on this psalm together with Jesus' words to His disciples in Matthew 9 verses 35-38:

[35]Jesus went through all the towns and villages, teaching in their synagogues, preaching the good news of the kingdom and healing every disease and sickness. [36]When He saw the crowds, He had compassion on them, because they were harassed and helpless, like sheep without a shepherd. [37]Then He said to his

disciples, "The harvest is plentiful but the workers are few. 38Ask the Lord of the harvest, therefore, to send out workers into his harvest field."

1   **Verse 5** *"Those who sow in tears"* and **verse 6** *"goes out weeping"* – meditate on the prerequisite feeling or condition of those who would engage in the service of God. Compare Matt. 9 v 36: Jesus *"had compassion on them, because they were harassed and helpless, like sheep without a shepherd."* Do you feel this compassion?

2   **Psalm 126 v 6a** *"carrying seed to sow"*
Meditate on those words and what they denote of work for God – e.g. the Gospel message or the ministry of healing. Compare Matt. 9 v 35: *"Jesus went through all the towns and villages, teaching in their synagogues, preaching the good news of the kingdom and healing every disease and sickness."*

3   **Psalm 126 v 6b** *"will return with songs of joy, carrying sheaves with him"* and **v 5** *"will reap with songs of joy".*
Meditate – compare Matt. 9 v 37: *"Then He said to his disciples, 'The harvest is plentiful but the workers are few'."* Meditate on the **certainty** of results in the end, because God blesses the work done in this way.
Meditate on the qualities a Christian worker must have, e.g. 'faithfulness' to result in "songs of joy" – God Himself rejoices over **one** sinner who repents – the result of the ministry of the pastor or evangelist.
Meditate on what these scriptures teach us about **real** Christian ministry.

Personal notes

A MEDITATION FOR THOSE WHO FEEL THAT GOD'S PRESENCE IS NOT WITH THEM – THAT HE IS ABSENT FROM THEIR LIVES

Psalm 139

[1]O LORD, You have searched me
and You know me.
[2]You know when I sit and when I rise;
You perceive my thoughts from afar.
[3]You discern my going out and my lying down;
You are familiar with all my ways.
[4]Before a word is on my tongue
You know it completely, O LORD.

[5]You hem me in — behind and before;
You have laid Your hand upon me.
[6]Such knowledge is too wonderful for me,
too lofty for me to attain.

[7]Where can I go from Your Spirit?
Where can I flee from Your presence?
[8]1f I go up to the heavens, You are there;
if I make my bed in the depths, You are there.
[9]If I rise on the wings of the dawn,
if I settle on the far side of the sea,
[10]even there Your hand will guide me,
Your right hand will hold me fast.
[11]If I say, "Surely the darkness will hide me
and the light become night around me,"

[12]even the darkness will not be dark to You;
the night will shine like the day,
for darkness is as light to You.
[13]For You created my inmost being;
You knit me together in my mother's womb.
[14]I praise You because I am fearfully and wonderfully made;
Your works are wonderful, I know that full well.
[15]My frame was not hidden from You
when I was made in the secret place.
When I was woven together in the depths of the earth,
[16]Your eyes saw my unformed body.
All the days ordained for me were written in Your book
before one of them came to be.
[17]How precious to me are Your thoughts, O God!
How vast is the sum of them!
[18]Were I to count them,
they would outnumber the grains of sand.
When I awake, I am still with You.
[19]If only You would slay the wicked, O God!
Away from me, you bloodthirsty men!
[20] They speak of You with evil intent;
Your adversaries misuse Your name.
[21]Do I not hate those who hate You, O LORD
and abhor those who rise up against You?
[22]I have nothing but hatred for them;
I count them my enemies.

[23]Search me, O God, and know my heart;
test me and know my anxious thoughts.
[24]See if there is any offensive way in me,
and lead me in the way everlasting.

1   **Verses 1-6**   *"O LORD, You have searched me and You know me.   You know when I sit and when I rise; You perceive my thoughts from afar.   You discern my going out and my lying down; You are familiar with all my ways.   Before a word is on my tongue You know it completely, O LORD. You hem me in – behind and before; You have laid Your hand upon me. Such knowledge is too wonderful for me, too lofty for me to attain."*
Meditate on the awesomeness of God's intimate and personal knowledge of you. "Such knowledge is too wonderful for me, too lofty for me to attain".

2   **Verses 7-12**   *"Where can I go from Your Spirit? Where can I flee from Your presence? 1f I go up to the heavens, You are there; if I make my bed in the depths, You are there. If I rise on the wings of the dawn, if I settle on the far side of the sea, even there Your hand will guide me, Your right hand will hold me fast.*

   "If I say, 'Surely the darkness will hide me and the light become night around me,' even the darkness will not be dark to You; the night will shine like the day, for darkness is as light to You."
Meditate on what theologians call the 'omnipresence of God' – thar He is everywhere at once – in heaven, the depths of the earth, all over the world – in the darkness as well as the light.

3   **Verses 13-18**   *"For You created my inmost being; You knit me together in my mother's womb. I praise You because I am fearfully and wonderfully made; Your*

works are wonderful, I know that full well. My frame was not hidden from You when I was made in the secret place. When I was woven together in the depths of the earth, Your eyes saw my unformed body. All the days ordained for me were written in Your book before one of them came to be. How precious to me are Your thoughts, O God! How vast is the sum of them! Were I to count them, they would outnumber the grains of sand. When I awake, I am still with You. If only You would slay the wicked, O God! Away from me, you bloodthirsty men!"

Meditation: God has always been in our lives – our fearful memories of the past can be healed by Him. He is with us night and day.

4   Verses 19-22 *"If only You would slay the wicked, O God! Away from me, you bloodthirsty men! They speak of You with evil intent; Your adversaries misuse Your name. Do I not hate those who hate You, O LORD, and abhor those who rise up against You? I have nothing but hatred for them; I count them my enemies."*

God will judge the wicked. As Christians we do not actually hate or abhor unbelievers, but this verse teaches that evil will not triumph over us.

5   Verse 23 *"Search me, O God, and know my heart; test me and know my anxious thoughts."*

Meditate on our exposure to God – of our anxious thoughts, or offensive ways. God will heal our innermost being, and lead us "in the way everlasting" – eternal life now, and for ever.

Personal notes

A MEDITATION FOR THOSE IN NEED OF GUIDANCE

Proverbs Chapter 3 verses 3-8

[3]Let love and faithfulness never leave you;
bind them around your neck,
write them on the tablet of your heart.
[4]Then you will win favour and a good name
in the sight of God and man.

[5]Trust in the LORD with all your heart
and lean not on your own understanding;
[6]in all your ways acknowledge Him,
and He will direct your paths.

⁷Do not be wise in your own eyes;
   fear the LORD and shun evil.
⁸This will bring health to your body
   and nourishment to your bones.

Although the Proverbs appear frequently as short pithy sayings, there is a theme which binds them together and this is true of the verses quoted here.

1 Verses 3-4   *"Let love and faithfulness never leave you; bind them around your neck, write them on the tablet of your heart. Then you will win favour and a good name in the sight of God and man."*

Meditate: love and faithfulness (reliability) are the hallmark of the man or woman who desires the guidance of God and fellow men and women. Meditate on what they mean to you and what part they have in your life.

2   Verse 4   *"Then you will win favour and a good name in the sight of God and man."*
Meditate – have you a "good name" and "favour" with God and your fellow men and women? What are they?

3   Verse 5 *"Trust in the LORD with all your heart and lean not on your own understanding"*
Meditate: what does it mean really to trust in the Lord? As you have a big decision to make, are you trying to work out what steps you should take in your life, are you trusting God, or trying to work it out yourself in your own mind?

4 **Verse 6** *"in all your ways acknowledge Him, and He will direct your paths."*
Meditate: what does it mean to acknowledge God in life's decisions or in the whole of one's life? You have to decide – are you going to direct your life, or are you putting it into God's hand: **abandoning** everything to Him and His leading. Only if we do the latter can we expect Him to guide us.

5 **Verses 7-8** *"Do not be wise in your own eyes; fear the LORD and shun evil. This will bring health to your body and nourishment to your bones."*
Meditate: here is more than the promise of guidance along life's path. If you reverence the Lord and shun evil you **are promised** the health and inner nourishment which are a by-product of a life that in all things puts God first, trusts Him and refers every decision to Him.

Personal notes

A MEDITATION FOR THOSE WHO FEAR THE FUTURE OF THE WORLD (1)

Isaiah Chapter 9 verses 1-7 and Chapter 11 verses 1-9

9: 1-7

[1]Nevertheless, there will be no more gloom for those who were in distress. In the past He humbled the land of Zebulun and the land of Naphtali, but in the future He will honour Galilee of the Gentiles, by the way of the sea, along the Jordan
[2]The people walking in darkness
have seen a great light;
on those living in the land of the shadow of death
a light has dawned.
[3]You have enlarged the nation
and increased their joy;
they rejoice before You
as people rejoice at the harvest,
as men rejoice when dividing the plunder.
[4]For as in the day of Midian's defeat,
You have shattered the yoke that burdens them,
the bar across their shoulders,

the rod of their oppressor.
[5]Every warrior's boot used in battle
and every garment rolled in blood
will be destined for burning,
will be fuel for the fire.
[6]For to us a child is born,
to us a son is given,
and the government will be on His shoulders.
And He will be called Wonderful Counsellor,
Mighty God, Everlasting Father, Prince of Peace.
[7]Of the increase of His government and peace
there will be no end.
He will reign on David's throne and over his kingdom,
establishing and upholding it with justice and righteousness
from that time on and for ever.
The zeal of the LORD Almighty will accomplish this.

11: 1-9

[1]A shoot will come up from the stump of Jesse;
from his roots a Branch will bear fruit.
[2]The Spirit of the LORD will rest on him –
the Spirit of wisdom and of understanding,
the Spirit of counsel and of power,
the Spirit of knowledge and of the fear of the LORD -
[3]and He will delight in the fear of the LORD.
He will not judge by what He sees with his eyes,
or decide by what He hears with his ears;
[4]but with righteousness He will judge the needy,
with justice He will give decisions for
the poor of the earth.
He will strike the earth with the rod of his mouth;

with the breath of his lips He will slay the wicked.
⁵Righteousness will be his belt
and faithfulness the sash round his waist.
⁶The wolf will live with the lamb,
the leopard will lie down with the goat,
the calf and the lion and the yearling together;
and a little child will lead them.
⁷The cow will feed with the bear,
their young will lie down together,
and the lion will eat straw like the ox.
⁸The infant will play near the hole of the cobra,
and the young child put his hand into the viper's nest.
⁹They will neither harm nor destroy
on all my holy mountain,
for the earth will be full of the knowledge of the LORD
as the waters cover the sea.

These words speak of the Perfect King, and who Jesus is in His glory.

Meditation: from these verses from Chapter 9 glean the following:

a) Verses 1-2 *"Nevertheless, there will be no more gloom for those who were in distress. In the past He humbled the land of Zebulun and the land of Naphtali, but in the future He will honour Galilee of the Gentiles, by the way of the sea, along the Jordan.*
The people walking in darkness have seen a great light; on those living in the land of the shadow of death a light has dawned."
Meditation: His rule is not only over Jews but also Gentiles and the whole world.

b) Verses 3-6 *"You have enlarged the nation and increased their joy; they rejoice before You as people rejoice at the harvest, as men rejoice when dividing the plunder.*
For as in the day of Midian's defeat, You have shattered the yoke that burdens them, the bar across their shoulders, the rod of their oppressor. Every warrior's boot used in battle and every garment rolled in blood will be destined for burning, will be fuel for the fire.
For to us a child is born, to us a son is given, and the government will be on His shoulders. And He will be called Wonderful Counsellor, Mighty God, Everlasting Father, Prince of Peace."
Meditation: The kingdom of God is inward – in the hearts of men and women as they **now** submit to God's rule.

c) *"Wonderful Counsellor"* – Jesus' perfect wisdom in His rule.

d) *"Mighty God"* – His absolute power – **now**.

e) *"Father"* – His everlasting care for His people.

f) *"Prince of Peace"* – His reign brings perfect peace to earth.

Glean from Chapter 11:

a) Verses 1-2 *"A shoot will come up from the stump of Jesse; from his roots a Branch will bear fruit. The Spirit of the LORD will rest on him – the Spirit of wisdom and of understanding, the Spirit of counsel and of power, the Spirit of knowledge and of the fear of the LORD –"*
Meditate on the Spirit of the Lord resting upon Him – compare

Luke 4: 14-21, *"Jesus returned to Galilee in the power of the Spirit, and news about Him spread through the whole countryside. He taught in their synagogues, and everyone praised Him.*
He went to Nazareth, where He had been brought up, and on the Sabbath day He went into the synagogue, as was His custom. And He stood up to read. The scroll of the prophet Isaiah was handed to Him. Unrolling it, He found the place where it is written:
'The Spirit of the Lord is on me,
because He has anointed me
to preach good news to the poor.
He has sent me to proclaim freedom for the prisoners
and recovery of sight for the blind,
to release the oppressed,
to proclaim the year of the Lord's favour.'
Then He rolled up the scroll, gave it back to the attendant and sat down. The eyes of everyone in the synagogue were fastened on Him, and He began by saying to them, 'Today this scripture is fulfilled in your hearing'."

b) Verse 2   Meditate on His discerning power.

c) Verse s 3-4a   *"and He will delight in the fear of the* LORD. *He will not judge by what He sees with his eyes, or decide by what He hears with his ears; but with righteousness He will judge the needy, with justice He will give decisions for the poor of the earth."*
This speaks of Divinely ordained equality.

d) Verses 4b-5   *"He will strike the earth with the rod of his*

93

mouth; with the breath of his lips He will slay the wicked. Righteousness will be his belt and faithfulness the sash round his waist."
This speaks of judgement.

e) Verses 6-9 *"The wolf will live with the lamb, the leopard will lie down with the goat, the calf and the lion and the yearling together; and a little child will lead them. The cow will feed with the bear, their young will lie down together, and the lion will eat straw like the ox. The infant will play near the hole of the cobra, and the young child put his hand into the viper's nest. They will neither harm nor destroy on all my holy mountain, for the earth will be full of the knowledge of the LORD as the waters cover the sea."*
How His eventual return as King Supreme will even affect nature.

Maranatha – Lord, come quickly.

Personal notes

A MEDITATION FOR THOSE NEEDING PEACE

Isaiah chapter 26 verses 3-4

[3]You will keep in perfect peace
him whose mind is steadfast,
because he trusts in You.
[4]Trust in the LORD for ever,
for the LORD, the LORD, is the Rock eternal.

1 Meditate on the word '**You**' – God – His power and His love. All you know about Him. All you have experienced of Him in your life.

2 Meditate on the word '**will**' – the absolute certainty – all you know of His promises in the Bible. He **never** breaks a promise.

3 Meditate on the word '**keep**' – the permanence of this promise of peace – it will never fluctuate.

4 Meditate on '**perfect peace**'. Imagine it – feel it – meditate until you have it.

5   Meditate on '**whose mind is steadfast**'. What does this mean for you – unshakable confidence.

6   Meditate on '**Because he trusts in You**'. Do you really trust God in your life and situation?   Meditate until you feel you trust Him absolutely.

7   Trust in the Lord '**for ever**'. Meditate until you have confidence that you will trust Him through all the changing circumstances of your life. Until you feel your trust will be with you for ever.

8   'The Lord is the **Rock eternal**'.   What does this mean for you? Security for ever. Meditate on this truth until you have really absorbed it into your mind and innermost being.

Personal notes

A MEDITATION FOR THOSE NEEDING INNER STRENGTH

Isaiah chapter 30 verse 15

This is what the Sovereign LORD,
the Holy One of Israel, says:
"In repentance and rest is your salvation,
in quietness and trust is your strength"

1   *'This is what the Sovereign Lord, the Holy One of Israel, says'.*
Meditate on what the **Sovereignty** of God means for you –
all-powerful – Ruler of the Universe – all humanity –
nothing is outside His control – He can meet all your needs.

2   *'the Holy One of Israel'*
Meditate on the **holiness** of God – absolute purity – before
which you are a sinner. Bring to Him any specific sins of your
life which come to your mind.

3   *'In repentance'*
Meditate on what **'repentance'** means – 'turning right
round', 'returning to God'– picture the return of the prodigal
son – picture yourself returning to God with all your being.

4   *'and rest'*
Really rest in the Lord – quieten your mind – "There is a place
of quiet rest near to the heart of God."

5 *'your salvation'*
Appropriate the salvation of your whole being: body, mind and spirit – 'salvation' really means 'being made whole'.

6 *'quietness and trust is your strength'*
Meditate on '**quietness**'– end of stress, confusion, anxiety and worry – feel the strength of the Sovereign loving God seeping into your whole being.

Personal notes

A MEDITATION FOR THOSE WHO ARE IN ANY WAY SICK

Isaiah chapter 53 verses 4-6 and 1 Peter 2 verse 24

[4]Surely He took up our infirmities
and carried our sorrows,
yet we considered Him stricken by God,
smitten by Him, and afflicted.
[5]But He was pierced for our transgressions,
He was crushed for our iniquities;
the punishment that brought us peace was upon Him,
and by His wounds we are healed.
[6]We all, like sheep, have gone astray,
each of us has turned to his own way;
and the LORD has laid on Him
the iniquity of us all.

1 Peter 2 verse 24: He himself bore our sins in his body on the tree, so that we might die to sins and live for righteousness; by his wounds you have been healed.

This passage from Isaiah is part of the most graphic prophecy foretelling our Lord's suffering and death upon the cross, foretold by Isaiah and repeated after the event by Peter in his first letter.

1   Verse 4   *"Surely He took up our infirmities and carried our sorrows, yet we considered Him stricken by God, smitten by Him and afflicted."*
Meditation: Are you in sorrow about anything which has

affected your life or the life of others? Then rejoice! Jesus is with you in your sorrow and has actually borne it in His death on the cross. **You need to feel it no more.** – Meditate until you feel it has been lifted from you by Jesus' suffering for you.

2   **Verse 5a**   *"But He was pierced for our transgressions, He was crushed for our iniquities"*
Do you feel any burden of sin or guilt? – Then be thankful – even joyful – Jesus has paid the price, has borne the suffering your sin deserved in Himself on the cross. Meditate until you have the assurance that this is absolutely true for you and the burden leaves you.

3   *"by His wounds we are healed"*
Meditate and picture the wounds – the bloodshedding of Jesus – the lashing of His back and legs by men using the lead-ended cords, the blood which flowed from His brow from the crown of thorns, the blood which flowed from His side when the spear was thrust in. Just as He has borne our iniquities and we need bear them no longer ourselves, so too He "took up our infirmities" (verse 4). So we likewise do not need to have these. Jesus took them away from us long ago by His suffering so that we no longer need to have them today or in the future. Enter into the healing Jesus won for you and appropriate it, just as you did for the forgiveness of your sins. Meditate until this is true for you.

Note: THERE IS HEALING FOR THE WHOLE PERSON
IN THE ATONEMENT.

Personal notes

A MEDITATION FOR THOSE WHO FEAR THE FUTURE (2)

Jeremiah chapter 29 verse 11

"For I know the plans I have for you," declares the LORD,
plans to prosper you and not to harm you,
plans to give you hope and a future."

Introduction: The Jewish nation had been defeated by the Babylonian armies and were exiles in Babylon, and (verse 2) "the king, the queen mother, the court officials, the leaders of Judah and Jerusalem, the craftsmen and the artisans had gone into exile from Jerusalem". They felt they had lost everything that really mattered to them and that their situation was hopeless; that they had no hope of their restoration. They had no real future. Jeremiah had been left in Jerusalem by the Babylonians, and from there he sent a letter (verse 4) to all those carried into exile, which contained the words of our meditation. These words were written under the inspiration of the Holy Spirit and can be appropriated by any one of God's people at any time for all times.

Meditation: *"for I know"* – Meditate on the one who knows – **God** – the all-powerful sovereign of the universe. He **knows** – there is **absolute certainty** in these words.

"the plans I have for you"
Meditate: **God** has a plan for your life – it is not victim to circumstances or chance, or in the hand of the evil one. This plan is for **you** – appropriate it now.

102

"plans to prosper you"
Meditate: your finances, your physical, mental and spiritual circumstances are going to be very good.

"not to harm you"
Meditate: God – who could – will not harm you or allow anything or anyone to do so.

"to give you hope"
Meditate – God will definitely give you hope – your situation is not in any way hopeless, no matter how you feel.

"and a future"
Meditate on the words of the song:

> I know who holds the future,
> And He will guide me with His hand;
> For **everything by Him is planned**.

Personal notes

A MEDITATION ON
THE LORD'S PRAYER

Matthew 6 verses 9-13

[9]This, then, is how you should pray:
Our Father in heaven,
hallowed be Your name
[10]Your kingdom come,
Your will he done
on earth as it is in heaven.
[11]Give us today our daily bread.
[12]Forgive us our debts,
as we also have forgiven our debtors.
[13]And lead us not into temptation,
but deliver us from the evil one.

1 *"Our"*
Meditate on the fact that this prayer is a corporate one, to be
used together by all God's children. **You never pray alone**
– always you are praying with other Christians somewhere.
Meditate on the fact that you **belong to a worldwide family**
of believers.

2 *"Father"*
Meditate on the astounding fact that, because of Jesus, you can

call the Creator of the universe "Father"! Meditate on all this means to you.

3 *"in heaven"*
Meditate – this is His address – where He abides, and that heaven is not somewhere above the sky, but is spiritually very close to you.

4 *"hallowed be Your name"*
Meditate on how **holy** God is and what this means to you.

5 *"Your kingdom come,*
Your will be done on earth as it is in heaven."
These two sentences are intertwined. Meditate on what God's kingdom means to you – in your life and daily living. Are you yourself living in the **will** of God?

6 *"Give us today our daily bread."*
Meditate: are you in financial need; do you get anxious about money? This petition is also **a promise** that the Father will provide for your basic needs.

7 *"Forgive us our debts"*
This means 'our sins'. Meditate – have you received assurance that all your sins are forgiven? Meditate until you are sure.

8 *"as we also have forgiven our debtors"*
Meditate – have **you** forgiven **everyone** living or dead who has sinned against you? Is there any resentment or bitterness in your heart?

9 *"And lead us not into temptation"*
Meditate: Are you undergoing temptation in any way − in
your mind, heart or soul? Ask God to help you overcome,
and return to this meditation until you have the victory.

10 *"but deliver us from the evil one"*
Meditation: All Christians are engaged in spiritual warfare
against Satan, 'the evil one'. Are you undergoing a real trial
and struggle against evil forces of darkness?   Meditate until
you are sure you have the victory.

Finish your meditation with an act of praise and adoration in the
words added in later manuscripts:

> For Yours is the kingdom and the power
> and the glory for ever.
> Amen.

Personal notes

A MEDITATION FOR THOSE WHO FEEL BURDENED

Matthew chapter 11 verses 25-30

[25]At that time Jesus said, "I praise You, Father, Lord of heaven and earth, because You have hidden these things from the wise and learned, and revealed them to little children. [26]Yes, Father, for this was Your good pleasure.

[27]All things have been committed to me by my Father. No one knows the Son except the Father, and no one knows the Father except the Son and those to whom the Son chooses to reveal Him. [28]"Come to me, all you who are weary and burdened, and I will give you rest. [29]Take my yoke upon you and learn from me, for I am gentle and humble in heart, and you will find rest for your souls. [30]For my yoke is easy and my burden is light."

Introduction. Imagine a familiar sight in Jesus' day – a yoke of oxen pulling a cart which is **very** heavy up a steep hill on a hot summer's day. They are straining; they are sweating. The driver is seated behind them, beating them to pull harder. Their feet keep slipping with the tremendous effort they are making. They become tired and weary but must keep going – keep pulling.

Meditation
1   Do you feel burdened like that? But must keep going on?

Are you burdened, say, with sin and guilt?

with failure?

with religious 'do's' and 'don'ts'?

with hurts?

with people – family, loved ones, an aged and sick parent or close relative for whom you have to care?

with bereavement?

with rejection?

with sickness – especially pain?

Don't try to ignore your burden. Really **feel it** at its worst. **Feel your weariness.**

2 Meditate on the great, unconditional invitation – **"COME TO ME."** Meditate on the Person, the love, the compassion of the One who invites you – He is gentle and humble in heart.

3 Come to Jesus – in your imagination and prayer – just where He stands – picture Him and come to Him.

4 What does it mean to "take **His** yoke upon you" in your prayer and daily life? – To learn from Him? **His** yoke is easy; **His** burden is light.

5 Now really relax and **feel the rest** He is giving to your body, mind and spirit. It is deep – "for your soul". Spend **a long time** feeling this rest, and do so with this meditation every day.

Personal notes

A MEDITATION FOR THOSE WHO FEEL BATTERED BY THE CIRCUMSTANCES OF LIFE

Mark chapter 4 verses 35-41

[35]That day when evening came, He said to his disciples, "Let us go over to the other side." [36]Leaving the crowd behind, they took Him along, just as He was, in the boat. There were also other boats with Him. [37]A furious squall came up, and the waves broke over the boat, so that it was nearly swamped. [38]Jesus was in the stern, sleeping on a cushion. The disciples woke Him and said to Him, "Teacher, don't you care if we drown?"

³⁹He got up, rebuked the wind and said to the waves, "Quiet! Be still!" Then the wind died down and it was completely calm. ⁴⁰He said to his disciples, "Why :ire you so afraid? Do you still have no faith'?"

⁴¹They were terrified and asked each other, "Who is this? Even the wind and the waves obey him!"

"A furious squall came up, and the waves broke over the boat, so that it was nearly swamped."
Meditation: In your imagination picture the scene – Jesus and the disciples in the midst of the Sea of Galilee. All is peaceful as they make their crossing to the other side of the sea. Suddenly a furious storm breaks loose. The waves are so high they are breaking over the boat and swamping it with water. Hear the wind. See the waves. Feel the absolute terror of the disciples as the boat will certainly, very soon sink. **Life can be like that** – all is well and peaceful – suddenly sickness, circumstances, situations we never expect hit us. We feel we are going under. We are terrified – there is nothing to cling on to. Is your life like that? Face it! **Feel** the desperation – the fear – even terror in your imagination.

"Jesus was in the stern, sleeping on a cushion. The disciples woke Him and said to Him, 'Teacher, don't you care if we drown?' "
Jesus is asleep – tired from all His day's teaching and ministry – sleeping through it all.
Meditation: Picture Jesus now – is He at the present time seemingly asleep – careless about your situation – not giving heed to your desperate plight – **doesn't He care?**

"He got up, rebuked the wind and said to the waves,

'Quiet! Be still!' Then the wind died down and it was completely calm."
Meditation: Jesus does care – **things are never out of His control**. He only has to speak into the situation – your situation – and there is a great calm.

"He said to His disciples, 'Why are you so afraid? Do you still have no faith?' "
Meditation: He speaks to the storm raging in the disciples' hearts. He rebukes them for lack of faith in God – in Him. Meditate until you have faith that He is in control – and keep on doing so until your panic and fear are gone and there is peace in your heart.

Personal notes

A MEDITATION FOR THOSE WHO FEEL OPPRESSED OR EVEN POSSESSED BY THE EVIL POWERS OF THE DEVIL

The healing of a demon-possessed man

Mark 5 verses 1-20

¹They went across the lake to the region of the Gerasenes. ²When Jesus got out of the boat, a man with an evil spirit came from the tombs to meet him. ³This man lived in the tombs, and no one could bind him any more, not even with a chain. ⁴For he had often been chained hand and foot, but he tore the chains apart and broke the irons on his feet. No one was strong enough to subdue him. ⁵Night and, day among the tombs and in the hills he would cry out and cut himself with stones.

,⁶When he saw Jesus from a distance, he ran and fell on his knees in front of Him. ⁷He shouted at the top of his voice, "What do you want with me, Jesus, Son of the Most High God? Swear to God that you won't torture me!" ⁸For Jesus had said to him, "Come out of this man, you evil spirit!" ⁹Then Jesus asked him, "What is your name?" "My name is Legion," he replied, "for we are many." ¹⁰And he begged Jesus again and again not to send them out of the area. ¹¹A large herd of pigs was feeding on the nearby hillside. ¹²The demons begged Jesus, "Send us among the pigs; allow us to go into them." ¹³He gave them permission, and the evil spirits came out and went into the pigs. The herd, about two thousand in number, rushed down the steep bank into the lake and were drowned.

[14]Those tending the pigs ran off and reported this in the town and countryside, and the people went out to see what had happened. [15]When they came to Jesus, they saw the man who had been possessed by the legion of demons, sitting there, dressed and in his right mind; and they were afraid. [16]Those who had seen it told the people what had happened to the demon-possessed man and told about the pigs as well. [17]Then the people began to plead with Jesus to leave their region. [18]As Jesus was getting into the boat, the man who had been demon-possessed begged to go with Him. [19]Jesus did not let him, but said, "Go home to your family and tell them how much the Lord has done for you, and how He has had mercy on you." [20]So the man went away and began to tell in the Decapolis` how much Jesus had done for him. And all the people were amazed.

Verses 1-5 *"They went across the lake to the region of the Gerasenes. When Jesus got out of the boat, a man with an evil spirit came from the tombs to meet Him. This man lived in the tombs and no one could bind him any more, not even with a chain. For he had often been chained hand and foot, but he tore the chains apart and broke the irons on his feet. No one was strong enough to subdue him. Night and day among the tombs and in the hills he would cry out and cut himself with stones."*

Meditate on the terrible condition of this man. Could anyone – you – be more in bondage to the devil than he was?

Verses 6-7 *"When he saw Jesus from a distance, he ran and fell on his knees in front of Him. He shouted at the top of his voice, 'What do you want with me, Jesus, Son of the*

Most High God? Swear to God that you won't torture me!' "
Meditation: See how the demons in the man recognised Jesus –
who He was – His power and authority over them. The same is
true for you.

Verse 8   *"For Jesus had said to him,   'Come out of this
man, you evil spirit!' "*
Meditate on how Jesus dealt with evil forces.

Verse 9   *"Then Jesus asked him, 'What is your name?'
'My name is Legion,' he replied, 'for we are many'."*
Meditation: Notice again how Jesus is totally in command of the
situation. This is also true for you.

Verse 10-15   *"And he begged Jesus again and again not
to send them out of the area. A large herd of pigs was
feeding on the nearby hillside. The demons begged Jesus,
'Send us among the pigs; allow us to go into them.' He gave
them permission, and the evil spirits came out and went into
the pigs. The herd, about two thousand in number, rushed
down the steep bank into the lake and were drowned.*

*"Those tending the pigs ran off and reported this in the
town and countryside, and the people went out to see what
had happened. When they came to Jesus, they saw the
man who had been possessed by the legion of demons,
sitting there, dressed and in his right mind"*
Meditate: Jesus completely delivers this man – He will also free
you if you completely trust Him and ask Him to do it. There is no
condition, qualification needed or anything else for you to do.

Verses 18-20   *"As Jesus was getting into the boat, the man*

114

who had been demon-possessed begged to go with Him. Jesus did not let him, but said, 'Go home to your family and tell them how much the Lord has done for you, and how He has had mercy on you.' So the man went away and began to tell in the Decapolis how much Jesus had done for him. And all the people were amazed."

Meditate on how it is important for you to testify about what Jesus has done for you so that His name will be glorified.

Closing thought:

The seventy-two returned with joy and said, "Lord, even the demons submit to us in Your name."

Jesus' authority over demons is now also delegated to His Spirit-anointed servants.

Personal notes

A MEDITATION FOR THOSE WITH PHYSICAL AFFLICTIONS.

The Woman who Was Bleeding to Death.

Mark 5 verses 21-43

[21]When Jesus had again crossed over by boat to the other side of the lake, a large crowd gathered around Him while he was by the lake. [22]Then one of the synagogue rulers, named Jairus, came there. Seeing Jesus, he fell at His feet [23]and pleaded earnestly with Him, "My little daughter is dying. Please come and put your hands on her so that she will be healed and live." [24]So Jesus went with him.

A large crowd followed and pressed around Him. [25]And a woman was there who had been subject to bleeding for twelve years. [26]She had suffered a great deal under the care of many doctors and had spent all she had, yet instead of getting better she grew worse. [27]When she heard about Jesus, she came up behind Him in the crowd and touched his cloak, [28]because she thought, "If I just touch his clothes, I will be healed." [29]Immediately her bleeding stopped and she felt in her body that she was freed from her suffering.

[30]At once Jesus realised that power had gone out from Him. He turned around in the crowd and asked, "Who touched my clothes?"

[31]"You see the people crowding against you," his disciples answered, "and yet you can ask, 'Who touched me?' "

---

^{32}But Jesus kept looking around to see who had done it. ^{33}Then the woman , knowing what had happened to her, came and fell at his feet and, trembling with fear, told Him the whole truth. ^{34}He said to her, "Daughter, your faith has healed you. Go in peace and be freed from your suffering."

^{35}While Jesus was still speaking, some men came from the house of Jairus, the synagogue ruler. "Your daughter is dead," they said. "Why bother the teacher any more?"

^{36}Ignoring what they said, Jesus told the synagogue ruler, "Don't be afraid; just believe."

^{37}He did not let anyone follow Him except Peter, James and John the brother of James. ^{38}When they came to the home of the synagogue ruler, Jesus saw a commotion, with people crying and wailing loudly. ^{39}He went in and said to them, "Why all this commotion and wailing? The child is not dead but asleep." ^{40}But they laughed at Him.

After He put them all out, He took the child's father and mother and the disciples who were with Him and went to where the child was. ^{41}He took her by the hand and said to her, "Talitha koum!" (which means "Little girl, I say to you, get up!") ^{42}Immediately the girl stood up and walked around (she was twelve years old). At this they were completely astonished. ^{43}He gave strict orders not to let anyone know about this, and told them to give her something to eat.

Meditation:
1. Imagine the scene: Jesus has crossed the lake and is by the side of the water. A large crowd had gathered around Him and was pressing in on Him. The disciples also were there near to Him, trying to keep the crowd from crushing Him on that lovely, sunny day. Then Jairus appears and Jesus is on His way to heal Jairus's

dying daughter when suddenly, Mark focuses on a nameless woman. Capture the scene as vividly as you can.

2. Now **imagine you are the woman.** Feel her desperate state — tried doctors — now without any money — getting worse — dying. Meditate until you feel 'in her shoes'.

3. She had heard about Jesus — His power to heal. Meditate on **all** you know **about Jesus** — on the Person of Jesus — picture Him as you imagine his physical person to be: what He looks like to you — His look of compassion.

4. Meditate on this woman's faith — not 'maybe', 'I hope', but "I will be healed". Continue in meditation until you have that faith.

5. She **touched** the outer part of His garments. In your imagination meditate until **you** feel you have touched the Risen Presence of Jesus who is present with you.

6. **Feel** that you are healed. Keep meditating until you, like her, feel healing from Jesus — **His power** flowing into you.

7. Hear His voice speaking to you: "Your faith has set you free from your affliction."

(**Advice**: use this meditation **slowly** and **frequently**.)

Personal notes

A MEDITATION ON THE PURPOSE JESUS HAS FOR OUR LIVES

Luke Chapter 4 verses 16-21

16He went to Nazareth, where He had been brought up, and on the Sabbath day He went into the synagogue, as was his custom. And He stood up to read. 17The scroll of the prophet Isaiah was handed to Him. Unrolling it, He found the place where it is written:
18"The Spirit of the Lord is on me,
because He has anointed me
to preach good news to the poor.
He has sent me to proclaim freedom for the prisoners
and recovery of sight for the blind,
to release the oppressed,
19to proclaim the year of the Lord's favour."
20Then He rolled up the scroll, gave it back to the attendant and sat down. The eyes of everyone in the synagogue were fastened on Him, 21and He began by saying to them, "Today this scripture

is fulfilled in your hearing."

In this passage Jesus lays His claim to be the Messiah. He has undergone His baptism in the Jordan when He was anointed by the Holy Spirit. He has emerged victorious from His temptations in the desert and now, at Nazareth, He sets out the whole panorama of what the programme and purpose of His ministry is to be.

Meditation:

1   Verse 18a   *"The Spirit of the Lord is on me, because He has anointed me to preach good news to the poor."*
This does not only mean the materially poor but also the 'poor in spirit' (see Matt. 5 v 3) which we all, by nature, actually are.   Meditate on how spiritually destitute you are without Jesus,   and then on the good news that all your sins are forgiven; you   have eternal life **now**; and you have been filled with the Holy   Spirit.

2   Verse 18b   *"freedom for the prisoners"*
Meditation: This does not only mean those who are literally in prison or captives through war,   but also those who are held captive, in bondage to anything, involving the spirit, mind or body. Meditate on anything that this is true of you – and **feel** the release Jesus brings to you.

3   Verse 18c   *"recovery of sight for the blind"*
It means what it literally says, as we see in Jesus' giving sight to the blind in His ministry. However, it includes every disability and every sickness which you may have. Meditate until you have appropriated this healing power.

4   Verse 18d   *"to release the oppressed"*

Again this is to be taken literally – e.g. all who are politically oppressed or oppressed in any way by other humans. However it also includes all who are oppressed in spirit, mind, or body by any force outside themselves, including Satanic opp-ression. Meditate until you feel the release Jesus brings deep in your being.

5 **Note:**

"Jesus Christ is the same yesterday and today
and for ever."

(Hebrews 13 v 8)

Personal notes

A MEDITATION FOR THOSE WHO FEEL THEY HAVE SINNED GREATLY

Luke Chapter 7 verses 36-50

[36]Now one of the Pharisees invited Jesus to have dinner with him, so He went to the Pharisee's house and reclined at the table. [37]When a woman who had lived a sinful life in that town learned that Jesus was eating at the Pharisee's house, she brought an alabaster jar of perfume, [38]and as she stood behind Him at his feet weeping, she began to wet his feet with her tears. Then she wiped them with her hair, kissed them and poured perfume on them.

[39]When the Pharisee who had invited Him saw this, he said to himself, "If this man were a prophet, he would know who is touching him and what kind of woman she is — that she is a sinner."

[40]Jesus answered him, "Simon, I have something to tell you."

"Tell me, teacher," he said.

[41]"Two men owed money to a certain money-lender. One owed him five hundred denarii and the other fifty. [42]Neither of them had the money to pay him back, so he cancelled the debts of both. Now which of them will love him more?"

[43]Simon replied, "I suppose the one who had the bigger debt cancelled."

"You have judged correctly," Jesus said.

[44]Then He turned towards the woman and said to

Simon, "Do you see this woman? I came into your house. You did not give me any water for my feet, but she wet my feet with her tears and wiped them with her hair. [45]You did not give me a kiss, but this woman, from the time I entered, has not stopped kissing my feet. [46]You did not put oil on my head, but she has poured perfume on my feet.

[47]Therefore, I tell you, her many sins have been forgiven — for she loved much. But he who has been forgiven little loves little."

[48]Then Jesus said to her, "Your sins are forgiven."

[49]The other guests began to say among themselves, "Who is this who even forgives sins?"

[50]Jesus said to the woman, "Your faith has saved you; go in peace."

1   **Verse 36**   *"Now one of the Pharisees invited Jesus to dinner with him, so He went to the Pharisee's house and reclined at the table."*
Imagine the scene – a dinner party – **for men only**. Imagine the room and the men "reclined at the table" awaiting food.

2   **Verse 37**   *"When a woman who had lived a sinful life in that town learned that Jesus was eating at the Pharisee's house, she brought an alabaster jar of perfume."*
Imagine – suddenly, uninvited a woman bursts in "who had lived a sinful life" – probably prostitution – not having committed just some sins but a **totally sinful life**.

3   **Verse 38**   *"and as she stood behind Him at his feet weeping, she began to wet his feet with her tears. Then she wiped them with her hair, kissed them and poured*

perfume on them."
Imagine this woman and enter completely into what she did to
Jesus. The perfume would be very costly, no doubt bought
with the proceeds of prostitution.
Meditate: **It represented her whole sinful life**. You can
bring your life, with its sin, to Jesus' feet in your imagination.
Do it!

4   **Verse 39**   *"When the Pharisee who had invited Him saw
this, he said to himself, 'If this man were a prophet, he
would know who is touching him and what kind of
woman she is – that she is a sinner'."*
Meditate: Jesus **did** know that she was a sinner, yet accepted
her offering – He will accept the offering of **your life.**

5   **Verses 40-43**   *"Jesus answered him, 'Simon, I have
something to tell you.' 'Tell me, teacher,' he said.
" 'Two men owed money to a certain money-lender.
One owed him five hundred denarii, and the other fifty.
Neither of them had the money to pay him back, so he
cancelled the debts of both. Now which of them will love
him more?' Simon replied, 'I suppose the one who had
the bigger debt cancelled.' 'You have judged correctly,'
Jesus said.*
Meditate on how much you love Jesus.

6   **Verses 44-47**   *"Then He turned towards the woman and
said to Simon, 'Do you see this woman? I came into
your house. You did not give me any water for my feet,
but she wet my feet with her tears and wiped them with
her hair. You did not give me a kiss, but this woman,*

from the time I entered, has not stopped kissing my feet. You did not put oil on my head, but she has poured perfume on my feet. Therefore, I tell you, her many sins have been forgiven – for she loved much. But he who has been forgiven little loves little'."

Meditate: Simon took Jesus for granted – how easy it is to do this. Do you?

7 **Verse 48** *"Then Jesus said to her, 'Your sins are forgiven'."*

Meditate and hear Jesus say to you, "Your sins are forgiven". Appropriate this into your very being.

8 **Verses 49-50** *"The other guests began to say among themselves, 'Who is this who even forgives sins?' Jesus said to the woman, 'Your faith has saved you; go in peace'."*

Hear these words and meditate upon them
and "Go in peace" from your meditation.

Personal notes

A MEDITATION FOR THOSE WHO HAVE GONE FAR AWAY FROM GOD AND WONDER IF THERE IS A POSSIBILITY OF RESTORATION

Luke Chapter 15 verses 11-32

[11]Jesus continued: "There was a man who had two sons. [12]The younger one said to his father, 'Father, give me my share of the estate.' So he divided his property between them.

[13]"Not long after that, the younger son got together all he had, set off for a distant country and there squandered his wealth in wild living. [14]After he had spent everything, there was a severe famine in that whole country, and he began to be in need. [15]So he went and hired himself out to a citizen of that country, who sent him to his fields to feed pigs. [16]He longed to fill his stomach with the pods that the pigs were eating, but no one gave him anything.

[17]"When he came to his senses, he said, 'How many of my father's hired men have food to spare, and here I am starving to death! [18]I will set out and go back to my father and say to him: "Father, I have sinned against heaven and against you. [19]I am no longer worthy to be called your son; make me like one of your hired men".' [20]So he got up and went to his father.

"But while he was still a long way off, his father saw him and was filled with compassion for him; he ran to his son, threw his arms around him and kissed him. [21]The son said to him, 'Father, I have sinned against heaven and against you. I am no longer worthy to be called your son.'

[22]"But the father said to his servants, 'Quick! Bring the best robe and put it on him. Put a ring on his finger and sandals on his feet. [23]Bring the fattened calf and kill it. Let's have a feast and

celebrate. [24]For this son of mine was dead and is alive again; he was lost and is found.' So they began to celebrate.

[25]"Meanwhile, the older son was in the field. When he came near the house, he heard music and dancing. [26]So he called one of the servants and asked him what was going on. [27]'Your brother has come,' he replied, 'and your father has killed the fattened calf because he has him back safe and sound.'

[28]"The older brother became angry and refused to go in. So his father went out and pleaded with him. [29]But he answered his father, 'Look! All these years I've been slaving for you and never disobeyed your orders. Yet you never gave me even a young goat so I could celebrate with my friends. [30]But when this son of yours who has squandered your property with prostitutes comes home, you kill the fattened calf for him!'

[31]" 'My son,' the father said, 'you are always with me, and everything I have is yours. [32]But we had to celebrate and be glad, because this brother of yours was dead and is alive again; he was lost and is found'."

Meditation:

1   Using your imagination picture the scene in the house – its magnificence and wealth, the servants, the father and the two brothers; and outside, the fields where there is growth of the crops. Then imagine you are the younger son asking for your share of the inheritance, and feel the large sum of money being given to you. Hold it – put it in your leather bag, and go out of the house. Put your belongings and the bag of money in your chariot and drive your horse to a far-off country.

2   Still as the younger son, imagine your life of luxury – your (illusory) sheer enjoyment of wild living (apart from the hangovers; fights and fear of having your money stolen).

3   Now imagine your life as the severe famine hits the country where you are.   You now have no money left and you are destitute – starving to death.

4   Now imagine yourself feeding the pigs (pigs were 'unclean' animals to a Jew, and to be a swineherd was the **very lowest** state into which a Jew could fall – the "scum of the earth"). Feel your pangs of intense hunger, so bad you would even eat the pigs' food.

5   Feel yourself getting so low that you come to your senses and in an act which would involve ultimate humiliation you decide to go home and fling yourself on your father's mercy – even willing to be counted no longer a son but a servant. Begin your long journey home.

6   " 'But while he was still a long way off, his father saw him and was filled with compassion for him; he ran to his son, threw his arms around him and kissed him'." Almost in astonishment, hear your father's words of forgiveness, feel his arms around you and his kiss.

7   **Verses 22-24**   " 'But the father said to his servants, "Quick! Bring the best robe and put it on him. Put a ring on his finger and sandals on his feet. Bring the fattened calf and kill it. Let's have a feast and celebrate. For this son of mine was dead and is alive again; he was lost and   is found." So they began to celebrate'." Feel the wonder of **complete restoration to sonship.** Meditate on what this teaches you about:

a)   Free will to leave God and the riches of His family and of being a **son.**

b) The abject result of sin and the condition into which it can get you.

c) Repentance.

d) God's graciousness.

e) Restoration to sonship.

8   Now imagine you are the elder brother – with a definitely valid point of view: " *'The older brother became angry and refused to go in. So his father went out and pleaded with   him. But he answered his father, 'Look! All these years I've been slaving for you and never disobeyed your   orders. Yet you never gave me even a young goat so I   could celebrate with my friends.   But when this son of yours who has squandered your property with prostitutes comes home, you kill the fattened calf for him!' "* and meditate on the father's reply to you: " *'My son,' the father said, 'you are always with me, and everything I have is yours'.* " and what it teaches of the blessings available to those who stay faithful to your Father-God.

Closing thought:

> In the same way, I tell you, there is rejoicing
> in the presence of the angels of God
> over one sinner who repents.

Luke 15 v 10)

Personal notes

A MEDITATION FOR WHOLENESS

John chapter 2 verses 1-11

[1]On the third day a wedding took place at Cana in Galilee. Jesus' mother was there, [2]and Jesus and his disciples had also been invited to the wedding. [3]When the wine was gone, Jesus' mother said to Him, "They have no more wine."

[4]"Dear woman, why do you involve me?" Jesus replied, "My time has not yet come."

[5]His mother said to the servants, "Do whatever he tells you."
[6]Nearby stood six stone water jars, the kind used by the Jews for ceremonial washing, each holding from twenty to thirty gallons.
[7]Jesus said to the servants, "Fill the jars with water," so they filled them to the brim.

[8]Then he told them, "Now draw some out and take it to the master of the banquet."
They did so, [9]and the master of the banquet tasted the water that had been turned into wine. He did not realise where it had come from, though the servants who had drawn the water knew. Then he called the bridegroom aside [10]and said, "Everyone brings out the choice wine first and then the cheaper wine after the guests have had too much to drink; but you have saved the best till now."
[11]This, the first of his miraculous signs, Jesus performed at Cana in Galilee. He thus revealed his glory, and his disciples put their faith in Him.

Meditation:

1 In your imagination picture the scene – the house – the crowd – the bride and bridegroom – the 'best man'. Feel the joy and happiness. Wedding celebrations at that time went on for several days. Picture Jesus, His mother and His disciples joining in.

2 *"Jesus and his disciples had also been invited to the wedding."* Reflection: Have you **invited Jesus** into your life and every circumstance of your life? If not, **do it!** Or if so, do it again – invite Him into this meditation.

3 *"They have no more wine."*
A serious eventuality – a need had arisen. Meditate on your need occurring even in the midst of your usual happiness.

4 *"Do whatever He tells you" " 'Fill the jars with water'."*
Reflect: Do you obey Him in everything without question when you are **sure** it is His will? Meditate on your obedience

to Jesus – even when it doesn't seem to make sense.

5   *"and the master of the banquet tasted the water that had been turned into wine"*
    Meditate on the **transforming presence of the Person of Jesus**. What else did He transform in His ministry e.g. sickness, the cross and the tomb.

6   Meditate on **what you need Jesus to transform in your life**. Continue to meditate until you believe He can do it, and come back to this meditation until He has done it.

7   Meditate on the fact that when Jesus transforms – then the **end result is better than it ever was before**.

Personal notes

A MEDITATION ON INTERCESSORY PRAYER FOR THE SICK

Introduction: In intercessory prayer we come to God in Christ for someone who is absent from us.

John chapter 4 verses 46-53

[46]Once more He visited Cana in Galilee, where He had turned the water into wine. And there was a certain royal official whose son lay sick at Capernaum. [47]When this man heard that Jesus had arrived in Galilee from Judea, he went to Him and begged Him to come and heal his son, who was close to death. [48]"Unless you people see miraculous signs and wonders," Jesus told him, "you will never believe." [49]The royal official said, "Sir, come down before my child dies." [50]Jesus replied, "You may go. Your son will live."

The man took Jesus at his word and departed. [51]While he was still on the way, his servants met him with the news that his boy was living. [52]W hen he enquired as to the time when his son got better, they said to hint, "The fever left him yesterday at the seventh hour." [53]Then the father realised that this was the exact time at which Jesus had said to him, "Your son will live." So he and all his household believed.

1   *"Once more He visited Cana in Galilee, where He had turned the water into wine. And there was a certain royal official whose son lay sick at Capernaum.   When this*

man heard that Jesus had arrived in Galilee from Judea, he went to Him and begged Him to come and heal his son, who was close to death."

Meditate on the love – the **compassion** which brought this royal official to Jesus on behalf of his son. Compassion is the prerequisite for intercessory prayer.

2 " *'Unless you people see miraculous signs and wonders,' Jesus told him, 'you will never believe'."*

At first Jesus seems to hesitate to grant this request. Meditate on times when Jesus seems to have delayed to grant your prayer.

3 *"The royal official said, 'Sir, come down before my child dies'."*

Meditate on the heartfelt cry and persistence of the nobleman.

4 *"Jesus replied, 'You may go. Your son will live.' The man took Jesus at his word and departed. While he was still on the way, his servants met him with the news that his boy was living."*

Meditate on the **power** of Jesus' spoken word and the **faith** with which it was received. Jesus speaks His word of healing now from His throne on high – today, and miracles happen – today.

5 *"When he enquired as to the time when his son got better, they said to him, 'The fever left him yesterday at the seventh hour'."*

6 *"Then the father realised that this was the exact time at which Jesus had said to him, 'Your son will live.' So he and all his household believed."*

Meditate on the way in which answered prayer brings glory to Jesus and belief in His Lordship.

Personal notes

A MEDITATION FOR THOSE WHO ARE PHYSICALLY ILL OR DISABLED

John chapter 5 verses 1-15

[1]Some time later, Jesus went up to Jerusalem for a feast of the Jews. [2]Now there is in Jerusalem near the Sheep Gate a pool, which in Aramaic is called Bethesda and which is surrounded by five covered colonnades. [3]Here a great number of disabled people used to lie – the blind, the lame, the paralysed. [5]One who was there had been an invalid for thirty-eight years. [6]When Jesus saw

him lying there and learned that he had been in this condition for a long time, he asked him, "Do you want to get well?"

[7]"Sir," the invalid replied, "I have no one to help me into the pool when the water is stirred. While I am trying to get in, someone else goes down ahead of me."

[8]Then Jesus said to him, "Get up! Pick up your mat and walk." [9]At once the man was cured; 'he picked up his mat and walked.

The day on which this took place was a Sabbath, [10]and so the Jews said to the man who had been healed, "It is the Sabbath; the law forbids you to carry your mat."

[11]But he replied, "The man who made me well said to me, 'Pick up your mat and walk'."

[12]So they asked him, "Who is this fellow who told you to pick it up and walk?"

[13] The man who was healed had no idea who it was, for Jesus had slipped away into the crowd that was there.

[14]Later Jesus found him at the temple and said to him, "See, you are well again. Stop sinning or something worse may happen to you." [15]The man went away and told the Jews that it was Jesus who had made him well.

Meditation:

1 Imagine the terrible scene – the pool – the five covered colonnades – the scene in the morning as a great number of disabled people are lying there – the blind, the lame, the paralysed – all with eyes fixed on the stagnant water, for it was believed that when the water in the pool bubbled, the first person to get into the pool would be healed.

2 Meditation: Now imagine that you are the invalid who has been in that condition for thirty-eight years. Then you see a

Rabbi – Jesus – coming towards you. You hear him say, "Do you want to get well?" You describe your dreadful predicament and say, "Sir, I have no one to help me into the pool when the water is stirred. While I am trying to get in, someone else goes down ahead of me."

3   Meditation: Hear Jesus say, "Get up! Pick up your mat and walk." Feel strength and power flowing into your legs, and in wonderment find that at once you are cured! You pick up your mat and walk.

4   Hear the controversy – the verbal accusations levelled against the man who healed you because you are carrying your mat on the Sabbath Day. Jesus has slipped away into the crowd.

5   Later Jesus finds you again. Hear Him say, "See, you are well again. Stop sinning or something worse may happen to you."

6   Now start excitedly telling everyone that it was Jesus who made you well.
      Meditate on the power of Jesus to heal even those who have been sick or an incurable invalid for a very long time – this includes you.
      Meditate on the fact that it was Jesus' spoken word that had the power to heal – hear Him speaking into your life, words – even commands – of healing.
      Meditate until you feel His healing power flowing into every part of your body.
      Meditate: Have you faith to **act** on Jesus' words.

      Meditate: on whether you **really** want to be well or have got conditioned, by being ill for a long time, to accept your illness and the idea that you cannot ever be healed.

Meditate: on the need for continual repentance to be well and keep well.

Personal notes

A MEDITATION FOR THOSE WHO FEAR DEATH

John chapter 11 verses 17, 21-27, 32-41

[17]On his arrival, Jesus found that Lazarus had already been in the tomb for four days.

[21]"Lord," Martha said to Jesus, "if you had been here, my brother would not have died. [22]But I know that even now God will give you whatever you ask."
[23]Jesus said to her, "Your brother will rise again."
[24]Martha answered, "I know he will rise again in the resurrection at the last day."
[25]Jesus said to her, "I am the resurrection and the life. He who believes in me will live, even though he dies; [26]and whoever lives and believes in me will never die. Do you believe this?"
[27]"Yes, Lord," she told him, "I believe that you are the Christ, the Son of God, who was to come into the world."

[32]When Mary reached the place where Jesus was and saw Him, she fell at his feet and said, "Lord, if you had been here, my brother would not have died."
[33]When Jesus saw her weeping, and the Jews who had come along with her also weeping, He was deeply moved in spirit and troubled. [34]"Where have you laid him?" He asked.
"Come and see, Lord," they replied.
[35]Jesus wept.
[36]Then the Jews said, "See how he loved him!"
[37]But some of them said, "Could not he who opened the eyes of the blind man have kept this man from dying?"

[38]Jesus, once more deeply moved, came to the tomb. It was a cave with a stone laid across the entrance. [39]"Take away the stone," He said.

"But, Lord," said Martha, the sister of the dead man, "by this time there is a bad odour, for he has been there four days."

[40]Then Jesus said, "Did I not tell you that if you believed, you would see the glory of God?"

[41]So they took away the stone. Then Jesus looked up and said, "Father, I thank You that You have heard me."

Verse 39   " 'Take away the stone,' He said. 'But, Lord,' said Martha, the sister of the dead man, 'by this time there is a bad odour, for he has been there four days'."
Meditation: Imagine you are Mary and Martha – they are in mourning – very distraught – yet they have a vague belief that their brother will rise again on the last day of world history. Feel their sadness with them. Feel their doubt – their brother has been dead four days – **he is very dead**.

Verses 25-26   "Jesus said to her, 'I am the resurrection and the life. He who believes in me will live, even though he dies; and whoever lives and believes in me will never die'."
Meditate on this amazing promise. 'I AM' is the Old Testament name of God: 'YAHWEH'. Meditate on the fact that eternal life is promised without doubt to all who **believe** in Jesus. Do you really believe in Him? Are you linked with His Person through faith? **Are you one with Him?**

Verses 43-44   "When He had said this, Jesus called in a loud voice, 'Lazarus, come out!' The dead man came *out, his hands and feet wrapped with strips of cloth, and a cloth around his face."*

Meditate: Jesus' promise is not mere words. In the raising of Lazarus **He demonstrated His power over death** – for Himself and all who believe in Him.

Meditate on this awesome power over man's final and, humanly speaking, invincible enemy.

Meditate: Seeing that Jesus has this tremendous power, is He not able to meet all your present needs? Bring them to Him, especially your fear of death, until you fear it no more.

Personal notes

A MEDITATION FOR THOSE WHO MINISTER DIVINE HEALING TO THE SICK

Acts 3 verses 1-16

[1]One day Peter and John were going up to the temple at the time of prayer — at three in the afternoon. [2]Now a man crippled from birth was being carried to the temple gate called Beautiful, where he was put every day to beg from those going into the temple courts. [3]When he saw Peter and John about to enter, he asked them for money. [4]Peter looked straight at him, as did John. Then Peter said, "Look at us!" [5]So the man gave them his attention, expecting to get something from them.

[6]Then Peter said, "Silver or gold I do not have, but what I have I give you. In the name of Jesus Christ of Nazareth, walk." [7]Taking him by the right hand, he helped him up, and instantly the man's feet and ankles became strong. [8]He jumped to his feet and began to walk. Then he went with them into the temple courts, walking and jumping, and praising God. [9]When all the people saw him walking and praising God, [10]they recognised him as the same man who used to sit begging at the temple gate called Beautiful, and they were filled with wonder and amazement at what had happened to him.

[11]While the beggar held on to Peter and John, all the people were astonished and came running to them in the place called Solomon's Colonnade. [12]When Peter saw this, he said to them: "Men of Israel, why does this surprise you? Why do you stare at us as if by our own power or godliness we had made this man walk? [13]The God of Abraham, Isaac and Jacob, the God of our

fathers, has glorified His servant Jesus. You handed Him over to be killed, and you disowned Him before Pilate, though he had decided to let Him go. [14]You disowned the Holy and Righteous One and asked that a murderer be released to you. [15]You killed the author of life, but God raised Him from the dead. We are witnesses of this. [16]By faith in the name of Jesus, this man whom you see and know was made strong. It is Jesus' name and the faith that comes through Him that has given this complete healing to him, as you can all see.

1   **Verses 1-2**   *"One day Peter and John were going up to the temple at the time of prayer – at three in the afternoon. Now a man crippled from birth was being carried to the temple gate called Beautiful, where he was put every day to beg from those going into the temple courts."*
Picture the scene in your imagination – a large number of Jewish men making their way to the temple through the 'Beautiful Gate' to pray – at three in the afternoon. Peter and John were amongst them. Outwardly they looked no different from anyone else going there. Picture the man, "crippled from birth", sitting there – a strategic place, holding out his begging bowl, asking for pity for his condition and charitable gifts from those entering through the gate.

2   **Verses 3-5** *"When he saw Peter and John about to enter, he asked them for money. Peter looked straight at him, as did John. Then Peter said, 'Look at us!' So the man gave them his attention, expecting to get something from them."*
The beggar asks Peter and John for money, but they **command** him to look intently at them. Meditate on why they

143

did this.

3   **Verses 6-10** *"Then Peter said, 'Silver or gold I do not have, but what I have I give you. In the name of Jesus Christ of Nazareth, walk.' Taking him by the right hand, he helped him up, and instantly the man's feet and ankles became strong. He jumped to his feet and began to walk. Then he went with them into the temple courts, walking and jumping and praising God. When all the people saw him walking and praising God, they recognised him as the same man who used to sit begging at the temple gate called Beautiful, and they were filled with wonder and amazement at what had happened to him."*
Meditate on what Peter and John did have – they carried within them the power of the Holy Spirit received on the Day of Pentecost. Meditate on the power of the Holy Spirit in your life every moment of day and night, which alone makes you essentially different from non-Christians, and gives you the power from God to heal. Imagine the scene described in these verses as if you were actually there.

4   *"While the beggar held on to Peter and John, all the people were astonished and came running to them in the place called Solomon's Colonnade. When Peter saw this, he said to them, 'Men of Israel, why does this surprise you? Why do you stare at us as if by our own power or godliness we had made this man walk? The God of Abraham, Isaac and Jacob, the God of our fathers, has glorified His servant Jesus. You handed him over to be killed, and you disowned him before Pilate, though he had decided to let him go. You dis-*

owned the Holy and Righteous One, and asked that a murderer be released to you. You killed the author of life, but God raised him from the dead. We are witnesses of this'."

Meditate on what Peter says to the crowd as the reason why they were able to heal this man.

5 **Verse 16** *"'By faith in the name of Jesus, this man whom you see and know was made strong. It is Jesus' name and the faith that comes through him that has given this complete healing'"*

Meditate on these words – especially on what authority is given you and the right to use Jesus' name. Also the importance of faith in His Name – which Peter and John have. Meditate ... until you are sure you have the power of the Holy Spirit within you and absolute faith in Jesus' Name – the two basic essentials for a Divine healing ministry.

Personal notes

A MEDITATION FOR WHOLENESS IN CHRIST JESUS

Ephesians chapter 1 and chapter 2 verses 1-8

[1]Paul, an apostle of Christ Jesus by the will of God,
To the saints in Ephesus, the faithful in Christ Jesus:
[2]Grace and peace to you from God our Father and the Lord Jesus Christ.
[3]Praise be to the God and Father of our Lord Jesus Christ, who has blessed us in the heavenly realms with every spiritual blessing in Christ. [4]For He chose us in Him before the creation of the world to be holy and blameless in His sight. In love [5]He predestined us to be adopted as His sons through Jesus Christ, in accordance with His pleasure and will — [6]to the praise of His glorious grace, which He has freely given us in the One He loves. [7]In Him we have redemption through His blood, the forgiveness of sins, in accordance with the riches of God's grace [8]that He lavished on us with all wisdom and understanding. [9]And He made known to us the mystery of His will according to His good pleasure, which He purposed in Christ, [10]to be put into effect when the times will have reached their fulfilment — to bring all things in heaven and on earth together under one head, even Christ.
[11]In him we were also chosen, having been predestined according to the plan of Him who works out everything in conformity with the purpose of His will, [12]in order that we, who

were the first to hope in Christ, might be for the praise of His glory. [13]And you also were included in Christ when you heard the word of truth, the gospel of your salvation. Having believed, you were marked in Him with a seal, the promised Holy Spirit, [14]who is a deposit guaranteeing our inheritance until the redemption of those who are God's possession – to the praise of his glory.

[15]For this reason, ever since I heard about your faith in the Lord Jesus and your love for all the saints, [16]I have not stopped giving thanks for you, remembering you in my prayers. [17]I keep asking that the God of our Lord Jesus Christ, the glorious Father, may give you the Spirit of wisdom and revelation, so that you may know Him better. [18]I pray also that the eyes of your heart may be enlightened in order that you may know the hope to which He has called you, the riches of His glorious inheritance in the saints, [19]and His incomparably great power for us who believe. That power is like the working of His mighty strength, [20]which He exerted in Christ when He raised Him from the dead and seated Him at His right hand in the heavenly realms, [21]far above all rule and authority, power and dominion, and every title that can be given, not only in the present age but also in the one to come. [22]And God placed all things under His feet and appointed Him to be head over everything for the church, [23]which is His body, the fulness of Him who tills everything in every way.

Chapter 2

[1]As for you, you were dead in your transgressions and sins, [2]in which you used to live when you followed the ways of this world and of the ruler of the kingdom of the air, the spirit who is now at work in those who are disobedient. [3]All of us also lived among

them at one time, gratifying the cravings of our sinful nature and following its desires and thoughts. Like the rest, we were by nature objects of wrath. [4]But because of His great love for us, God, who is rich in mercy, [5]made us alive with Christ even when we were dead in transgressions – it is by grace you have been saved. [6]And God raised us up with Christ and seated us with Him in the heavenly realms in Christ Jesus, [7]in order that in the coming ages He might show the incomparable riches of His grace, expressed in His kindness to us in Christ Jesus. [8]For it is by grace you have been saved, through faith – and this not from yourselves, it is the gift of God.

1   **Verse 4a**   *"For He chose us in Him before the creation of the world"*
Meditate on this truth – you are not in this world by chance – or even the desire of your parents. Your birth, **as a unique individual**, was planned by God before He set the sun ablaze.

2 **Verses 7-8a**   *"In Him we have redemption through His blood, the forgiveness of sins, in accordance with the riches of God's grace that He lavished on us"*
Meditation: Think of your sins – your failures in your life – He already made provision for them to be forgiven. Think of the cross – the blood of Christ – and meditate until you feel, you are sure – no spot of guilt remains in you.

3   **Verse 5a** *"He predestined us to be adopted as His sons"*
Meditate on this truth that you have been adopted by God as one of His precious children – a member of His family – an heir with Christ.

4   **Verses 13b-14a**   *"Having believed, you were marked in Him with a seal, the promised Holy Spirit, who is a deposit **guaranteeing** our inheritance"*
Meditate until you have received **assurance** that verse 7 and verse 5 are true for you and you are certain of your place in heaven.

5   **Verse 3b**   *"who has blessed us in the heavenly realms with every spiritual blessing in Christ."*
Meditate on what a wonderfully blessed person you are.

6   **Ch. 2 verse 6**   *"God raised us up with Christ and seated us with Him in the heavenly realms in Christ Jesus"*
Read Ch. 1 verses 20-23. Meditate on where Christ is now – then read Ch. 2 verses 1-5: where you were. Then meditate on where you are spiritually now – far above all demons and evil forces – feel your place of **victory**.

Personal notes

A MEDITATION FOR THOSE WHO FEEL THEIR FAITH IS WEAK

Ephesians chapter 3 verses 14-21

[14]For this reason I kneel before the Father, [15]from whom His whole family in heaven and on earth derives its name. [16]I pray that out of His glorious riches He may strengthen you with power through His Spirit in your inner being, [17]so that Christ may dwell in your hearts through faith. And I pray that you, being rooted and established in love, [18]may have power, together with all the saints, to grasp how wide and long and high and deep is the love of Christ, [19]and to know this love that surpasses knowledge – that you may be filled to the measure of all the fulness of God.

[20]Now to Him who is able to do immeasurably more than all we ask or imagine, according to His power that is at work within us, [21]to Him be glory in the church and in Christ Jesus throughout all generations, for ever and ever! Amen.

1   *"out of His glorious riches"*
     What are these? Think about them and meditate upon them.

2   *"that He may strengthen you ... in your inner being"*
     Do you need strength? Do you feel weak? Meditate upon "He" – **God** – and the strength He promises, until you **feel** it.

3   *"with power through His Spirit in your inner being"*

Meditate upon God's power. Feel His Spirit dwelling within you. Soak His power into your **inner** being – deep inside you and reaching every part of your being.

4 *"so that Christ may dwell in your hearts through faith"*
What a promise! Meditate upon it and the Christ of the Gospels – now risen – is actually dwelling within you if you have invited Him in – meditate on the promise – **He is there** in your innermost being.

5 *"may have power ... to grasp how wide and long and high and deep is the love of Christ, and to know this love that surpasses knowledge"*
Meditate until **you** know this love.

6 *"filled to the measure of all the fulness of God."*
Meditate until you feel **you** are filled with all this fulness.

7 *"Now to Him who is able"*
Meditate on God's power – He is **able** to meet your need.

8 *"to do immeasurably more than all we ask or imagine"*
What are you asking? Imagining? He can do even more. Meditate upon this truth.

9 *"according to His power that is at work within us"*
Meditate until you feel His power at work within you.

Personal notes

A MEDITATION ON SPIRITUAL WARFARE

Ephesians chapter 6 verses 10-18

[10]Finally, be strong in the Lord and in His mighty power.
[11]Put on the full armour of God so that you can take your stand against the devil's schemes. [12]For our struggle is not against flesh and blood, but against the rulers, against the authorities, against the powers of this dark world and against the spiritual forces of evil in the heavenly realms. [13]Therefore put on the full armour of God, so that when the day of evil comes, you may be able to stand your ground, and after you have done everything, to stand. [14]Stand

firm then, with the belt of truth buckled round your waist, with the breastplate of righteousness in place, [15]and with your feet fitted with the readiness that comes from the gospel of peace. [16]In addition to all this, take up the shield of faith, with which you can extinguish all the flaming arrows of the evil one. [17]Take the helmet of salvation and the sword of the Spirit, which is the word of God. [18]And pray in the Spirit on all occasions with all kinds of prayers and requests. With this in mind, be alert and always keep on praying, for all the saints.

Introduction: From the moment a person becomes a Christian he/she is immediately involved in spiritual warfare. The devil doesn't like to lose those who were his own, and tries to get them back under his sway. Also, throughout our Christian lives he and his minions try to attack a Christian's body, mind and spirit and his/her circumstances. As Paul says, ultimately our struggle is not against flesh and blood (human beings) but against authorities, against the powers of this dark world and against spiritual forces of evil (beings without bodies) in the heavenly places.

1 *"Therefore put on the full armour of God, so that when the day of evil comes, you may be able to stand your ground, and after you have done everything, to stand."*
Meditation: We cannot prevail against those powerful forces by ourselves. We need the power of God in our lives in order to triumph. We have, as our invincible help, the power of God Himself – His 'mighty power'. So we need not be in any way afraid. Whenever we feel under attack we must, in prayer, draw on the omnipotent power of God, and then we shall always 'stand' – BE TRIUMPHANT.

2 *"put on the full armour of God"*
   Meditation: Paul urges us to put on "armour", and he illustrates this by drawing on the battledress of a Roman soldier when we are attacked by the enemy, and then our Christian faith will remain intact.

3 *"the belt of truth"*
   Meditation: The devil is a liar from the beginning and tries to sow seeds of doubt in our minds. Jesus, however, said, "I am the truth" (John 14 v 6). So we take hold again of our Faith, which is the ultimate truth. In your imagination put on this belt – buckle it around your waist.

4 *"the breastplate of righteousness"*
   Meditation: This means the righteousness you have from faith in Jesus' death, resurrection and ascension which ensures that you are cleansed from all sin.   It also means 'right living' – complete obedience to Christ who is the 'Way' (John 14 v 6). In your imagination actually put it on to protect your heart and chest.

5 *"feet fitted with the gospel of peace"*
   Meditation: This peace comes from God as you live as far as is possible at peace with all people.

6 *"the shield of faith"*
   This is a metal shield, which covers the body from knees to chin.   The flaming arrows of the evil one absolutely cannot penetrate your complete faith in God and His Son Jesus – your trust in all He is and has done for you.   In your imagination

pick it up and place it in front of you.

7   *"the helmet of salvation"*
Meditation: You have been saved (Ephesians 2 v 8) from sin and guilt and all its consequences. The evil powers can find no way to knock you out with a blow to the head, as long as you accept this salvation as complete. In your imagination put this helmet on your head.

8   *"the sword of the Spirit"*
Meditation: This, Paul says, is "the word of God". You don't only defend yourself against the devil, you go on the attack by quoting at the evil powers the written word of God – texts you have learnt which you quote at him and his minions, as Jesus did in His temptations in the desert. When the devil attacked Him, He replied, "It is written ..." (Matthew 4). In your imagination take up this sword – know your Bible!

Concluding thought: There is no reason at all why a Christian should be overcome by the evil one as long as he/she takes these words to heart.

Personal notes

A MEDITATION ON PETITIONARY PRAYER

Philippians chapter 4 verses 6-8

Introduction: It is not wrong or selfish to pray asking God for anything which we need ourselves. In fact the Lord Jesus taught us that this is so in the Lord's Prayer, where one of the petitions is, "Give us today our daily bread". We should not hesitate therefore to make petitions for ourselves to our Heavenly Father. Paul teaches us how to do this in his letter to the Philippians, Chapter 4 verses 6-8:

[6]Do not be anxious about anything, but in everything, by prayer and petition, with thanksgiving, present your requests to

God. [7]And the peace of God, which transcends all understanding, will guard your hearts and your minds in Christ Jesus.

[8]Finally, brothers, whatever is true, whatever is noble, whatever is right, whatever is pure, whatever is lovely, whatever is admirable – if anything is excellent or praiseworthy – think about such things.

1   *Meditation:* Our prayers, worship and petitions should arise from **joy** in our hearts in, through, and **despite** our needs and circumstances. Right now, let your joy arise to your Lord Jesus.

2   *"Do not be anxious about **anything**, but in everything, by prayer and petition, with **thanksgiving**"*
Meditation: When we bring our cares and needs to God, they should arise not only from joy, but also from thanksgiving. Now! Thank God for all He has done for you in Jesus and in the whole of your past and present life. Write them down in your 'Personal notes' section.

3   *"present your requests to God"*
Meditation: List your needs in the 'Notes' section and make sure that you leave out **nothing** which you want God to do or give you and others.

4   *"And the peace of God, which transcends all understanding, will guard your hearts and your minds in Christ Jesus."*
Meditation: When we are really, **in faith**, believing God will answer, He will meet our every need: past, present and future. When we **really** believe this – then the peace of God, **which**

transcends all understanding, will guard (literally 'stand as a sentry') at the door of our hearts and minds.
Repeat this meditation until you **really** appropriate and **feel** that peace.

Personal notes

A MEDITATION FOR ALL WHO ARE AFRAID OR ANXIOUS ABOUT ANYTHING PAST, PRESENT OR FUTURE

1 Peter 5 verse 7

Cast all your anxiety on Him because He cares for you.

1   Meditate on anything or everything that is making you anxious or fearful. It is very helpful in this meditation if you actually write them down in the 'Notes' section.

2   Then cast each one upon the Lord.   The word 'cast' is the same one that is used for a fisherman casting his net into the sea. This means that you literally 'fling' your care upon the sea of God's infinite love for you.

3   Meditate upon the fact that God knows all about your personal individual cares and fears, for His knowledge of you is so intimate that He knows even the number of hairs on your head (Matthew 10 v 30).

4   Meditate on the nature of God – His infinite power and love – His very Being.   He can carry your own personal cares "because He cares for you" and is able to work **all** things you care about for a very good purpose and end (Romans 8 v 28).

5   Meditate on the fact that you have no need to have these cares, anxieties and fears burdening you, because you are a child of your infinite, powerful and loving Heavenly Father who can and will take very good care of you.

Personal notes

A MEDITATION FOR THOSE SUFFERING BEREAVEMENT

Introduction: You have lost a loved one or more than one. Where are your departed loved ones? Is it right to wish they were with you when we believe they are in heaven? **But is there really a heaven?** Can we be certain? If so, what is heaven like? It is difficult to imagine a life without time and space. What are they doing? The most vivid pictures of life in heaven are given in the book of Revelation. I will reproduce the relevant sections of that Book with little comment for guidance in meditation. The most important exercise for you to do is for you to use your imagination. Lift up your spirit and imagine the scenes – imagine you are in the vast throng of departed Christians – joined with your departed loved ones **who are actually there**.

Revelation 5 verses 6-end

[6]Then I saw a Lamb, looking as if it had been slain, standing in the centre of the throne, encircled by the four living creatures and the elders. He had seven horns and seven eyes, which are the seven spirits of God sent out into all the earth. [7]He came and took the scroll from the right hand of Him who sat on the throne. [8]And when He had taken it, the four living creatures and the twenty-four elders fell down before the Lamb. Each one had a harp and they were holding golden howls full of incense, which are the prayers of the saints. [9]And they sang a new song:

161

"You are worthy to take the scroll
and to open its seals,
because You were slain,
and with Your blood You purchased men for God
from every tribe and language and people and nation.
[10]You have made them to be a kingdom
and priests to serve our God,
and they will reign on the earth."

[11]Then I looked and heard the voice of many angels, numbering thousands upon thousands, and ten thousand times ten thousand. They encircled the throne and the living creatures and the elders. [12]In a loud voice they sang:
"Worthy is the Lamb, who was slain,
to receive power and wealth
and wisdom and strength
and honour and glory and praise!"
[13]Then I heard every creature in heaven and on earth and under the earth and on the sea, and all that is in them, singing:
"To Him who sits on the throne and to the Lamb
be praise and honour and glory and power,
for ever and ever!"
[14]The four living creatures said, "Amen", and the elders fell down and worshipped.

Meditation: Join in the praise and worship – actually sing the praise as best you can. Notice the central, dominating Person is that of Jesus, bearing still the marks of the wounds of His crucifixion.

Revelation 7 verses 9-end

[9]After this I looked and there before me was a great multitude that no one could count, from every nation, tribe, people and language, standing before the throne and in front of the Lamb. They were wearing white robes and were holding palm branches in their hands. [10]And they cried out in a loud voice:

"Salvation belongs to our God,
who sits on the throne,
and to the Lamb."

[11]All the angels were standing round the throne and around the elders and the four living creatures. They fell down on their faces before the throne and worshipped God, [12]saying:

"Amen!
Praise and glory
and wisdom and thanks and honour
and power and strength
be to our God for ever and ever.
Amen!"

[13]Then one of the elders asked me, "These in white robes – who are they, and where did they come from?"

[14]I answered, "Sir, you know."

And he said, "These are they who have come out of the great tribulation; they have washed their robes and made them white in the blood of the Lamb.
[15]Therefore,

"they are before the throne of God
and serve Him day and night in His temple;
and He who sits on the throne
will spread His tent over them.

^{16}Never again will they hunger;
never again will they thirst.
The sun will not beat upon them,
nor any scorching heat.
^{17}For the Lamb at the centre of the throne
will be their shepherd;
He will lead them to springs of living water.
And God will wipe away every tear from their eyes."

Meditation: Now notice the condition of absolute bliss of those in heaven – imagine it – enter into it.

Revelation 21 verses 1-7

^{1}Then I saw a new heaven and a new earth, for the first heaven and the first earth had passed away, and there was no longer any sea. ^{2}I saw the Holy City, the new Jerusalem, coming down out of heaven from God, prepared as a bride beautifully dressed for her husband. ^{3}And I heard a loud voice from the throne saying, "Now the dwelling of God is with men, and He will live with them. They will be His people, and God Himself will be with them and be their God. ^{4}He will wipe every tear from their eyes. There will be no more death or mourning or crying or pain, for the old order of things has passed away."

^{5}He who was seated on the throne said, "I am making everything new!" Then He said, "Write this down, for these words are trustworthy and true."

^{6}He said to me: "It is done. I am the Alpha and the Omega, the Beginning and the End. To him who is thirsty I will give to drink without cost from the spring of the water of life. ^{7}He who overcomes will inherit all this, and I will be his God and he will be my son."

Meditation: This is a picture of the Lord God's ultimate, final, absolute life for all believers. Enter into it – it is one vast family.

"He who overcomes [endures all that life on earth can do to them] ***will*** *inherit all this, and I will be his God and he will be my son."*

Enter into and rejoice at where your departed loved ones are in fact **right now**.

Personal notes

A MEDITATION ON HOW TO BE AN OVERCOMER

Introduction: The Bible teaches that in this Age of Grace the devil is allowed to assail Christians in many ways. This freedom that Satan has will end at the Second Coming of our Lord Jesus Christ, when the evil one and all his minions will be cast into the "lake of fire". In the meantime we must learn to be overcomers, as the devil can attack our spirit with doubts and fears, our minds with depression and other mental disorders, and our bodies with pain and sickness. The following verse from Revelation teaches how we can, in fact, overcome all his assaults.

Revelation chapter 12 verse 11

They overcame him
by the blood of the Lamb
and by the word of their testimony;
they did not love their lives so much
as to shrink from death.

1 Meditate on *"the blood of the Lamb"*.
This means Jesus' sacrificial death on the cross. A hymn writer wrote of the "Blood of Jesus":

Oft as it is sprinkled
On our guilty hearts
Satan in confusion
Terror-struck departs.

166

(18th Century author unknown)

2 Meditate on the word of your testimony. This means your out-
spoken declaration of your experience of your salvation and
all that Jesus has done for you.

3 Meditate on the words: *"they did not love their lives so
much as to shrink from death."*
This means, in the words of Paul (Romans 12 v 1) that you
have already become a "living sacrifice" – meditate on what
this means for you. Dying the death of a martyr would, if
needed, be the absolutely definite consequence of the fact that
you are "already dead" and "your life is hidden with Christ in
God" (Colossians 3 v 3).

If these three factors are true of you, then the Bible says you will
be an overcomer.

Personal notes

Conclusion

I hope that you have read this book from beginning to end, selecting those topics that speak to you. If so you will have learnt a great deal about what the Bible teaches concerning wholeness through Jesus Christ. If, as I hope, you have **meditated** on **every one** of these topics and made notes as to what God has said to you, then you will have a treasury of devotion to which you can return whenever you feel in need of spiritual enrichment.

I have made no promise of instantaneous healing results, although from past experience these may well take place. If you have given God time and space in your life, then I believe the LIVING AND ACTIVE WORD OF GOD will be at work in your whole being, bringing spiritual growth and healing and wholeness. You will have been like a pleasure boat sailing around an island, constantly bringing on board your life rich spiritual treasure, without ever taking your spiritual eyes from the island itself, the Word of God.

I will leave with you one final word from the Bible, which you should memorise and to which you should return repeatedly, for it is a profound and sure promise from God to you and every one of His faithful children, and is my personal prayer for you:

"May God Himself, the God of peace,
sanctify you through and through.
May your whole spirit, soul and body be kept blameless
at the coming of our Lord Jesus Christ.
The One who calls you is faithful and He will do it."
(! Thessalonians 5 v 23-24)

Appendix A

Some more verses that speak of healing
for you to memorise and appropriate for yourself

Psalm 30 v 2-3   O Lord my God, I called to You for help
and You healed me. O Lord, You brought me up from the
grave; You spared me from going down to the pit.

Psalm 147 v 3   He heals the broken-hearted and binds up
their wounds.

Isaiah 57 v 18-19   "I have seen his ways, but I will heal him;
I will guide him and restore comfort to him, creating praise on
the lips of the mourners in Israel. Peace, peace, to those far
and near," says the Lord. "And I will heal them."

Jeremiah 30 v 17   "But I will restore you to health and heal
your wounds," declares the Lord, "because you are called an
outcast, Zion for whom no one cares."

Jeremiah 17 v 14   Heal me, O Lord, and I shall be healed;
save me and I shall be saved, for You are the one I praise.

Isaiah 58 v 8   Then your light will break forth like the dawn,
and your healing will quickly appear; then your righteousness
will go before you, and the glory of the Lord will be your rear
guard.

Hosea 14 v 4   "I will heal their waywardness and love them freely, for My anger has turned away from them."

Matthew 4 v 23   Jesus went throughout Galilee, teaching in their synagogues, preaching the good news of the kingdom, and healing every disease and sickness among the people.

Matthew 8 v 16   When evening came, many who were demon-possessed were brought to Him, and He drove out the spirits with a word and healed all the sick.

Matthew 9 v 35   Jesus went through all the towns and villages, teaching in their synagogues, preaching the good news of the kingdom and healing every disease and sickness.

Matthew 12 v 15   Aware of this, Jesus withdrew from that place. Many followed Him, and He healed all their sick.

Matthew 15 v 30   Great crowds came to Him, bringing the lame, the blind, the crippled, the mute and many others, and laid them at his feet; and He healed them.

Joshua 1 v 5   "No one will be able to stand up against you all the days of your life. As I was with Moses, so I will be with you; I will never leave you nor forsake you."

Matthew 28 v 20b   "And surely I am with you always, to the very end of the age."

Mark 1 v 34   and Jesus healed many who had various diseases. He also drove out many demons, but He would not let the demons speak because they knew who He was.

James 5 v 15 And the prayer offered in faith will make the sick person well; the Lord will raise him up. If he has sinned, he will be forgiven.

Romans 8 v 11 And if the Spirit of Him who raised Jesus from the dead is living in you, He who raised Christ from the dead will also give life to your mortal bodies through His Spirit, who lives in you.

John 14 v 13 "And I will do whatever you ask in my name, so that the Son may bring glory to the Father."

John 15 v 7 "If you remain in me and my words remain in you, ask whatever you wish, and it will be given you."

John 14 v 27 "Peace I leave with you; my peace I give you. I do not give to you as the world gives. Do not let your hearts be troubled and do not be afraid."

Mark 11 v 24 "Therefore I tell you, whatever you ask for in prayer, believe that you have received it, and it will be yours."

Appendix B

The following is an abbreviated testimony of a lady who had obviously meditated and reflected long and hard on the account of the raising of Lazarus. She held on to this even though her condition grew worse. In the end the Word triumphed and broke through, and she was miraculously healed.

Testimony as published in *The Pattern*, September 1960.

THE STORY OF MY
MIRACULOUS HEALING

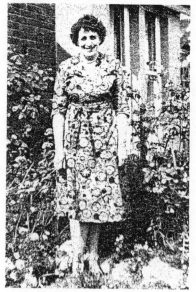

By

MRS MARGERY
STEVEN

(as recorded for broadcasting over I.B.R.A. Radio)

On July 4th, 1960, Jesus healed me miraculously, and only His nail-pierced hand touched me.
To tell you about this wonderful miracle I must first go back to my childhood. When I was about 6 years of age, my father was very ill with a spinal complaint; in fact doctors felt he would do no more work, but through the manager of his place of employment my mother and father were taken to Bournemouth to see Principal George Jeffreys who was conducting a revival and healing campaign in a large Tent there in the year 1926. Through the preaching of the Word, which I sincerely believe from cover to cover, both my parents were converted. To me, this is the most wonderful miracle of all, greater than healing of the body, for when Jesus changes the heart and life so many marvellous things can happen.

My father also received a healing touch from the Lord through the laying on of hands and the anointing with oil by God's servant, Principal George Jeffreys, in the same campaign in 1926, and this enabled him to return to his job of engineering for the next 18 years. To God be all the glory!

This wonderful healing touch established in me, as a little girl, a faith in God and I sincerely believed, as I do now, that Jesus Christ is the same yesterday, and today, and forever.

Because of the conversion of my parents they sent me to Church and Sunday School. I do thank God for my Sunday School teachers, for they faithfully told me the Bible stories week by week; but out of all they told me the one thing that lived for me was the raising of Lazarus from the dead, as recorded in St. John's Gospel, chapter 11. I know my Lord was preparing me away back in those early days, for He knew of the 5½ years' illness I would have to suffer and that the miracle of Lazarus would live for me.

[Having worked as a nurse, including in a military hospital in

the Second World War, she continues:] All that ended, however, 5 years ago. Following a trying illness, multiple sclerosis, or creeping paralysis, attacked me before I realised it. I first began to fail generally, then to lose power in a leg or arm, and then my sight became affected. But God's promise remained: "My grace is sufficient for thee: for My strength is made perfect in weakness."
Gradually I got worse, until 20 months ago I became so helpless as my legs became useless, that I had to be lifted from bed to wheel-chair, like a baby, and strapped around with belts to keep me from falling forward. Often my parents fed me as I had no control over the spoon with which I tried to feed myself. The food was cut up by my mother as I had no power in my left arm. My left eye was completely closed, my right eye often had treble vision, so I had to wear dark glasses to try to help the sight of that eye.

About eight months ago I started to have blackouts when I would lose consciousness for hours, but still with all this Jesus Himself had implanted faith in his Word, and I used to say to my dear Christian friends: "What my Lord could do for Lazarus, He can do for me if it is His will."

Things got worse for me. Then on February 4th of this year I dreamed :during the night that I was sitting in a chair by my bed (as when I was fit enough my father and mother would lift me there from my bed so that my mother would be able to wash me more easily). As I dreamed I thought I put out my left leg, then I awoke to find it was a dream. Then a voice sounded through my room — it was my Lord's, in these words: "Tarry a little longer."
In the next few days I told several of my praying friends about the way I had received this message from Jesus in the night whilst I was alone with Him. From that moment my faith became stronger, although I got slowly worse in health until my speech was also so badly affected that at times I could not make myself

understood. But in all this suffering was the realisation — what Jesus could do for Lazarus He could do for me! And His message to me to tarry a little longer meant that in His own good time He would heal me. I left the future to Him; it did not seem to matter if it took days or years for my Lord to deliver me, for I knew He would in the end.

On Monday, July 4th, exactly five months after God had spoken to me, my Lord healed me, in the very chair of which I had dreamed! I had said goodbye to my husband at five minutes to six on that Monday morning — a helpless woman. At 6.15 my mother gave me a cup of tea. At 6.20 my father and mother lifted me from my bed, strapped me in the chair beside the bed, put a bell in my good hand, to summon aid if needed, and left me alone. Mother went to get my washing water and my father had gone to get a towel from upstairs. Then in a matter of seconds, when I was all on my own, my Lord Jesus healed me! I felt a warm glow go over my body. My left foot, which was doubled up, straightened out; my right foot, the toes of which were pointed towards my heel, came back into position. I grasped the handle of my bedroom door which was beside me, undid the straps which were about my body, and said, "By faith I will stand," which I did. With that I thought of my mother and the shock it would be to her if she came back to find her daughter standing after so many years, so I sat down and called for her. With that both my parents came running to my room, thinking I was in need of them. I said, "Mum dear, take my hands, please don't be afraid, something wonderful has happened." I. put out my right arm and as I did so my left arm came out from behind me and joined the other! It was so wonderful a few minutes afterwards to find I could wear my own wedding ring, which I had not been able to do for years, as my fingers of that hand had got so thin. My mother said, "Darling, how wonderful, your hand is warm, and is well again." I said, "Mum, dear, it's more wonderful than that. I can stand." With that, holding her hands, I stood once more on my two feet. Then, gently putting my parents to one side, I said "Dears, I don't need your help any more, I'm walking with God." Unaided I then walked from my bedroom, through the small dining room to the kitchen, my parents following mutely behind me. When I reached the kitchen I turned and went hack into the dining room and, taking off. my glasses, I said, "Mum, I can trust God for my hands and feet. I can trust Him for my sight." With that, in a moment, my left eye opened and my sight was fully restored! In fact Jesus made such a perfect job I do not need the glasses I had before I was ill and I am now writing dozens of letters a day! To Him be all the glory!

I felt that I wanted this testimony to be such that people would forget Margery Steven and think of and thank her Lord only for the great things He has done.

We told no one until I had been examined by my doctor, and he confirmed the miracle on Tuesday, July 5th. Since then several doctors and nurses have been to see me, and they have gone away knowing that only God has wrought this wonderful miracle: so please, forget Margery Steven and remember WHAT JESUS ALONE CAN D0.

A comment by one of Margery's friends

My dear friends in Christ Jesus. You have just heard Margery's testimony. During her long illness I have cried, after seeing her poor twisted body, but also have come away marvelling at her wonderful faith in Christ Jesus. She used to quote to me "and by His stripes we are healed". He died on the cross to heal our bodies as well as to save our souls.

I went to visit Margery with a few flowers on July 6th, 1960, quite expecting to hear her mother say, "I'm afraid she is not well enough to see visitors today", as I knew she had been lapsing into unconsciousness for hours on end. Instead I was met at the door by the smiling face of her mother, who was her faithful nurse and companion through all the weary years of illness. She greeted me with the words, "Have you heard the news — I have some wonderful news." As I went into the front room, her mother told me of her daughter's healing. I was like Thomas, I doubted. It just would not register, a dying girl suddenly restored to health. It could not he possible.

Suddenly the door opened and Margery walked in. I was amazed, astonished, speechless, after the crippled body and the skeleton I knew. In its place I saw a tall well built woman with the aura of Christ about her. .We knelt and thanked God for this wondrous miracle. Praise His Holy Name! I rushed out of the house, stopping all my friends, telling the marvellous news.

Many people have come to know the Lord Jesus through Margery's testimony. She, like. Job, was tested unto death and yet she praised the Lord through it all. Dear friends, as you are reading this give your lives to Jesus today, and He will be as great a Friend to you as He was and is to Margery Steven.

M. M.

Index

Meditations:

General Index